U.S. Health Care and the Future Supply of Physicians

U.S. Health Care
and the
Future Supply
of Physicians

Eli Ginzberg
Panos Minogiannis

Transaction Publishers
New Brunswick (U.S.A.) and London (U.K.)

Library of Congress Catalog Number: 2003053134
ISBN: 0-7658-0198-1
Printed in the United States of America

Library of Congress Cataloging-in-Publication Data

Ginzberg, Eli, 1911-
    U.S. health care and the future supply of physicians / Eli Ginzberg and Panos Minogiannis.
        p. cm.
    Includes bibliographical references and index.
    ISBN 0-7658-0198-1 (cloth : alk. paper)
        1. Medical care—United States. 2. Medical policy—United States. 3. Physicians—Supply and demand—United States. 4. Health care reform—United States. I. Minogiannis, Panos. II. Title.

RA395.A3G567 2003
362.1'0973—dc21   2003053134

Contents

Introduction:
The Problem and Its Setting

This introduction will provide the reader with some critical insights into how this book came to be written; its sponsoring foundation; and the nature of the collaboration between the senior and the junior author. It will also elaborate on some defining characteristics such as the doubling of the U.S. population of the elderly by 2030 and the likely consequences of this development on the care and treatment of the much enlarged number of the chronically ill elderly whose numbers are expected to double from around 35 million to over 70 million.

A few markers of events starting in 1980: National Health Expenditures (NHE) for that year had risen to around $245 billion, up from $41 billion in 1965 when Medicare and Medicaid were first enacted. Ronald Reagan was elected president in November 1980 by a comfortable margin, but the country was entering a serious recession. After several decades of increases in the number of patients admitted to acute-care hospitals, the early 1980s saw a marked decline (about 20 percent), which was not recaptured in the following years except for the steep acceleration in the number of patients admitted and treated and discharged on the same day from the hospital.

With employers facing double-digit annual premium increases for their employee health insurance policies, the steep decline in inpatient hospital admissions in the early 1980s provided them an opportunity in selected market areas, such as Southern California, the Twin Cities, and a few other locations with large established managed-care arrangements to seek lower health insurance renewal rates in exchange for a higher number of enrollees. By the mid-to-late 1980s a considerable amount of new financing had become available to encourage the rapid growth of managed-care companies to a point where, by the early 1990s, the earlier long-term trend to double-digit increases in health insurance premiums had finally been arrested with most workers having been shifted out of fee-for-service coverage into an HMO or PPO arrangement.

But the end of the 1990s saw a rising discontent from both insured patients and their physicians. Many patients resented having to revisit their gatekeeper generalist physician before returning to their specialist who was overseeing one or more of their chronic illnesses and treatments; and more and more physicians resented having their decisions overridden by managed-care officials. By the late 1990s, many enrollees with the support of their physicians and with further support from their employers secured health insurance coverage that provided more freedom of choice to the enrolled even though it was slightly more costly. Managed-care plans suffered considerable drops in enrollments.[1]

In early 2000, the Eisenhower Center of Columbia University was informed by June Osborne, the recently appointed new president of the Josiah Macy Jr. Foundation, that the foundation trustees with whom the Eisenhower Center at Columbia University had had relations since the early 1970s, had granted our request for a year's support to prepare a volume on U.S. Health Care and the Future Supply of Physicians. My junior colleague, Panos Minogiannis, who completed his doctorate at Columbia's Mailman School of Public Health with special distinction before returning to his country, Greece, to complete his period of military service. His dissertation, entitled *European Integration and Health Policy: The Artful Dance of Economics and History,* was published by Transaction Publishers, New Brunswick, New Jersey, in 2003.[2]

The remainder of this introduction will deal first with the critical health policy issues that confronted the United States in the last decade of the twentieth century, and, secondly, will call attention to the challenges that the United States will confront by 2030 when the nation's elderly, those above 65 years of age, will have doubled from 35 to 70 million, with the predominate number living at home, many of whom will be suffering from one or more chronic illnesses.

At the beginning of the 1990s, the American Association of Medical Colleges launched a program, "3000 by 2000," which aimed to enlarge the number of students of African American background who were admitted to the nation's allopathic medical schools. Regrettably, after a good start, the program fell far short of its goals.

On the other hand, the underrepresentation of women in U.S. medicine, who as late as the latter 1960s accounted for no more than

8 percent of the nation's total number of physicians in training, had been almost totally eliminated with women accounting for almost 48 percent of the entrance class in 2002, a six-fold gain. Challenges remain with respect to an enlarged role for women physicians in leadership positions in academic medical centers, and the odds favor a slow but continuing correction.

For the better part of the two last decades, if not longer, the United States has confronted conflicting views about the appropriate proportions of generalists to specialists in training. At the peak of the managed-care expansion in the 1990s, the proportion of generalists in training increased but more recently the ratio has declined, and with more than 80 percent of the U.S. population urban based, the dominance of specialists is likely to continue.

The leadership of U.S. medicine—the AAMC, the AMA, the leaders of Osteopathic Medicine—have collectively advised Congress to cut back the number of foreign-born International Medical Graduates (IMGs) admitted under special immigration regulations to pursue residency training in the United States to no more than 10 percent of the number of U.S. graduates. However, to date Congress has not seen fit to follow this advice because of its awareness of the fact that IMGs treat disproportionate numbers of the under-served urban and rural low-income population that U.S. graduates tend to avoid.

In 1995, a PEW Commission on health personnel under the chairmanship of former Governor Lamm of Colorado recommended the closure of twenty U.S. medical schools by 2005, a recommendation that has been disregarded by all groups concerned with the future of U.S. health personnel.

As of the beginning of the twenty-first century, we have clear evidence that physicians are not playing more than a marginal role in looking after the chronic elderly patients living at home and there is little reason to anticipate any marked changes in the decades ahead in their practice mode. The bulk of the care that these patients require and receive comes from non-physician clinicians, primarily RNs, nurse practitioners, physician assistants, and selected non-physician therapists. Odds are that these groups will continue to provide most of the home-care services required by the chronically ill. Several challenges remain: the desirability of increasing the opportunities for physicians in training to share some training experiences with non-physician clinicians; the possibility that the United States will imitate the recently adopted innovation introduced by the German government to provide financial support for families that commit themselves to care for one or more homebound elderly; with the experiment expanded to include neighborhood daycare clinics for the care of many of the homebound.

The United States needs to take advantage of the larger part of the decade that remains to experiment with improved care for the about-to-double homebound chronically ill.

Notes

1.   These are the parameters that set the working environment for the nation's physicians. Admittedly, it is one of volatility and when one realizes that 14 percent of GDP is spent on health care, one has to wonder where that money goes and perhaps, more importantly, whether there are changes that can be introduced into the system in order to control the rise of expenditures. An area, perhaps the most important in which one could potentially intervene is in the supply of health care personnel. This has been one the long-term interests of the staff at the Eisenhower Center for the Conservation of Human Resources. Therefore, it is only fitting that the final project of the Center should focus on this subject.

2.   Prior to that, we collaborated fruitfully on a number of projects over a period of four years.

1

Why Focus on Physician Supply?

The simplest answer to the rhetorical question that provides the title to this opening chapter emphasizes that the availability of physicians is the key determinant of whether all of the nearby inhabitants in an area will be able to access a physician if and when they need to do so. A further point: since most physicians still continue to practice in the United States as independent practitioners, the decisions that they make about the diagnosis and treatments that their patients should receive affects both their own earnings as well as playing a key role in determining the expenditures of the health care sector. And thirdly, the manner in which physicians practice, solo or as members of a smaller or larger group of colleagues; office or hospital-based; in close association or not with a group of non-physician clinicians and medical technicians will determine to a marked degree the efficiency and effectiveness of the health care services that they provide to the patients who come to them for advice and treatment. In short, while many different sectors of our modern society, from government to health insurance companies, managed care organizations, academic health centers, the pharmaceutical industry and still other groups, exercise varying degrees of influence on how the nation's health care system operates with particular reference as to the availability of medical access for the population, to costs, and to the quality of the care provided, the physician remains the key to the efficiency and effectiveness of the health care services that the public receives. It is the licensed physician alone who is authorized by law to provide a wide range of treatments that, if mishandled, can result in injury or even to the premature death of the patient rather than to his or her recovery and future well-being.

Put differently, physician supply has historically been the approach to address larger questions that face U.S. health care policymakers.

These questions include: How can we provide equitable access? How can we provide quality care? How can we accomplish these ends within a reasonable cost? The centrality of the physician supply in the U.S. health care system is the connecting link to these broader questions. How many doctors we have, what kind, what ethnicity/ gender, from what schools, where they practice, how they practice— all these questions and many more are important because of their potential to affect the system's financing, access to it, and the delivery modes. This is why focusing on physician supply is important and this is why it should be studied within this broad context.

Looking back to the U.S. policy experience, there are three kinds of policies that have affected physician supply: (1) policies that directly targeted physician supply, (2) broader health care reforms, (3) other societal reforms. Furthermore, they have been initiated by both government and private sector as well as by the profession itself. A brief review of selective policy initiatives can be rewarding. It is by no means exhaustive, but nevertheless indicates that (1) there are many actors involved in this arena, and (2) their actions interact with one another, often in ways that would have been difficult to predict beforehand.

Policies That Target the Physician Supply

In the early-to-mid-1960s, more specifically between 1963 and 1965, the federal government took the lead to double the output of U.S. medical schools on the assumption that the 140 physicians per 100,000 population, the national ratio as of 1960, was grossly insufficient to meet the future needs of the American people, more specifically because of their increasing affluence and the steady advances that were being made by "high-tech" medicine with respect to diagnosis, treatment, and rehabilitation. After thirteen years of liberal federal funding, further increased by state and private sector funding, Congress declared in 1976 that the prior existing physician shortage had been eliminated. At that point, Congress appointed a Graduate Medical Education National Advisory Committee (GMENAC) to assess and report on future trends in the supply and specializations of U.S. physicians. In 1980 and 1981, after detailed studies to meet the Congressional charge, GMENAC reported that the United States would face in 1990 an excess of almost 70,000 physicians and by century's end an excess of 145,000—or of the order of 20 percent, too many physicians in the year 2000. Because of the recent assumption to office of the Reagan administration and the worsening recession, Washington paid little attention to the GMENAC report. What is more, most of the leading medical and medical educational organizations failed to take the report's findings seriously, among other reasons because the current health marketplace, despite the severe recession, had not led to any widespread underemployment much less unemployment of physicians or to any notable decline in their annual earnings. When academic studies are not confirmed by current economic trends their prognostications are likely to be ignored which was the experience of GMENAC.

Another example of a policy that directly targeted the physician supply was the earlier formation of the National Health Service Corps. Despite the substantial funding for the expansion of graduates from U.S. medical schools, and the further large-scale flow of federal and state funding to Medicare and Medicaid enrollees which further improved the financial well-being of most of the nation's acute care hospitals and enlarged the earnings of the nation's physicians, Congress recognized as early as 1970 that the large-scale expansion of the physician supply did not assure ready access to physician care for substantial numbers of the population located in "underserved areas." Consequently, Congress established the National Health Service Corps, which made special funding available to physicians and other scarce health care workers who were willing to relocate for a number of years to practice in underserved areas.

Broader Reforms

We need to look more closely at several other major departures in public policy during the critical three-year period (1963-65) that also influenced the number and types of physicians to be trained for future practice. In 1964, Congress passed the Civil Rights Bill, which initially addressed the removal of discrimination based on race, but to facilitate its passage the sponsors also outlawed discrimination based on gender. At the time of the bill's passage the United States had one of the lowest representation of women physicians among all of advanced nations in the world, under 10 percent; Spain alone ranked below the United States. At the end of the twentieth century, the number of women graduates from U.S. medical schools had risen over four-fold to over 40 percent of the current graduating class.

However, the impact of the 1964 legislation on the admission and graduation of "underrepresented minorities," primarily African Americans and Latinos, lagged far behind the rate of expansion for women, but still increased significantly. However, in 1991, when the American Association of Medical Colleges (AAMC) launched its new program of "3000 by 2000" (underrepresented minority graduates from U.S. medical schools), the program fell short of its goal, primarily because the number of qualified candidates applying for medical school during the course of the decade fell. Leaders of the underrepresented minorities as well as leaders of the medical profession saw significant gains from increased numbers of minority groups having the opportunity to be treated by physicians who shared their racial or ethnic backgrounds and would therefore be better positioned to diagnose and treat them. Faced with the anticipated explosive growth of the Hispanic population in the first third of the twenty-first century, the issue of increasing the number of medical students from underrepresented minorities must remain high on the nation's agenda.

Broader Health Care Reforms

Although the AMA withdrew its long-term opposition to direct federal financing for U.S. medical schools in 1963 in order to marshal its efforts more effectively to defeat a federally financed Medicare bill that was in the hopper, Congress ignored the AMA opposition and passed Medicare (and Medicaid) early in 1965. While the major goal of the legislation was to provide federal funding to enable much broader access for the elderly and the poor to the health care system, the new legislation had a major influence on the physician supply, not only by enabling more patients to seek and pay for their medical care, but further, Medicare made substantial new federal funding available to the academic medical centers and other teaching hospitals. The newly enacted Graduate Medical Education (GME) funding also increased the salary levels for residents in training. It enabled many of them to pursue specialist and subspecialty training that often extended their residency training to seven or eight years and even longer for a small minority.

Although Robert Ebert, former dean of Harvard Medical School, warned his colleagues that the explosive growth in the number of physicians in training to become specialists and subspecialists would provide direct competition for the leading medical centers they ignored his warning, among other reasons because they saw their future primarily as leaders in biomedical research and in providing high-tech medical treatments. With Medicare and Medicaid able to transform the financial outlook of many of the nation's hospitals from marginal to comfortable because of Medicare's reimbursement policy of cost/plus, together with reducing the number of patients who previously had been treated as charity patients, the leading Academic Health Centers (AHCs) continued to prepare a large number of specialists, many of whom started practices in the suburbs and helped to upgrade many suburban hospitals.

Another health care policy that was broader in nature but was affected by, and in turn itself affected the physician supply was the creation of community health centers. The establishment in the latter 1960s of federally funded and staffed community health centers aimed to respond to the special problems of underserved populations. And a further federal initiative dates from 1971 when federal dollars became available for starting family care residencies on the theory that many residents who would complete their training in low density regions would be more likely to start practices close to where they had been trained.

A third development that affected the broader health care environment and had direct effects on the types of physicians in training was the expansion of managed care. The employer community, especially in areas with a long experience with managed care arrangements, such as in Southern California and the Twin Cities and a few other locales, starting in the early 1980s, looked for ways to moderate the double-digit increases that they had experienced in their premium payments for providing their workers with health insurance coverage. Aided by a growing surplus of hospital beds reflecting the increasing shift from inpatient to ambulatory care for an increasing number of procedures, and further recognizing that a growing number of physicians were able, willing, and even anxious to fill their appointment schedules, new managed care companies, mostly for-profit, were able to obtain "discounts" from hospitals and physicians to whom they referred additional patients and to share their savings from such arrangements with employers who were able to switch their employees from fee-for-service coverage to one or another type of prepayment. The managed care company paid the participating physician a set fee to oversee the medical care needs of their patients by serving as a gatekeeper who had to approve ahead of time more costly requests such as consultations with specialists, expensive diagnostic procedures, admission to a hospital and the required length of stay, and still other decisions that had earlier been made by the patient and his or her physician. By the early-to-mid-1990s, the managed care companies had largely reversed the trend to ever higher premium rates and at the same time they were making good profits and paying their executives high salaries and bonuses. The rapid growth of managed care had the direct effect of creating an enlarged demand for generalist physicians. In more recent years, as we will see, the trend has reversed itself again as many managed care companies have found themselves in increasing turmoil.

Another reason for studying the physician supply is that during the closing decade of the twentieth century, we saw a number of additional physician supply issues emerge on the agendas of important and influential medical societies and leading health care centers. After more than a decade's neglect of GMENAC's findings about the coming large surplus of physicians, research reports by two leading health care analysts, David Kindig of the University of Wisconsin and Jonathan Wiener of Johns Hopkins in 1993 and 1994 published major articles that reopened the physician surplus issue. But once again, the trends in physician earnings, which did decline in 1994 but only in that year, failed to provide the confirmation that the leaders of the profession and the deans of the leading medical schools would have required to take the forecast of the coming surplus seriously and to look for ways to mitigate its potential bad effects.

It would be a mistake, however, to suggest that the medical leadership in the 1990s responded to the Kindig-Wiener analysis of a prospective large physician surplus in the same manner as the medical leadership had reacted to the comparable findings of GMENAC a decade earlier. By the early 1990s, a growing number of key professional medical groups had become concerned about the prospective surplus of physicians, at least to the point of considering a reduction in the large and growing numbers of foreign-born graduates of foreign medical schools (IMGs) who were being admitted for residency training in the United States, a high proportion of whom would eventually alter their immigration status to enable them to remain and practice in the United States. The data, as the century neared its end, revealed that IMGs accounted for just under 1:4 of all physicians in active practice.

In 1997, with the American Association of Medical Colleges and the AMA in the lead, together with support from other concerned professional groups, a conjoint statement was issued that Congress ought to take early action to reduce the numbers of IMGs by "limiting federal funds for GME positions." They concurred with COGME's recommendation that the number of IMGs be reduced from its recent levels of 25 to 30 percent of the graduates of U.S. medical schools to no more than 10 percent of the number of the 1993 U.S. medical school graduates.

Congress' unwillingness to act in response to this broad- based request of the leadership of organized medicine, as well as the medical educational leadership, can best be explained by the following. The concerned parties recognized that a significant proportion of IMGs at the beginning as well as at the completion of their residency training accepted positions in medical shortage areas that graduates of U.S. medical schools tended to shun. In fact, 95 percent of IMGs holding exchange visitor visas reported that they would be establishing practices in shortage areas. And, three-quarters of all physicians starting practices in shortage areas were IMGs. Further, IMGs accepted positions not only in shortage areas but also in safety-net hospitals in many locations that care for disproportionate numbers of uninsured and low-income patients. Moreover, in 1998, IMGs were broadly represented, at least initially, in the primary care specialties, with 49 percent training in family practice, internal medicine, pediatrics, preventive medicine, and geriatric medicine. Aware that even if many or most IMGs relocate after spending a period of years in an underserved area, Congress realized that if it reduced radically the numbers allowed to pursue residency training in this country, the care of patients in underserved areas would worsen, with little or no prospect that IMGs would be replaced by graduates of U.S. medical schools.

The question must therefore be asked and answered why, with fewer physicians being available to care for persons in underserved locations, the key professional medical organizations recommended that Congress reduce the number of IMGs to no more than 10 percent of the graduates of U.S. medical schools. The answer is not immediately obvious but the question is relevant, even if Congress has refused to date to act on it. The leaders of medical organizations are increasingly concerned that the United Stats faces a potential surplus of physicians with many believing that the surplus is already here and others believing that it will arrive shortly. In the face of this present and/or prospective surplus, medical leadership believes that a reduction in the number of IMGs admitted to the United States now is the best assurance that in the out years the number and output of U.S. medical schools will not have to be cut back.

But Congress has been reluctant to follow the advice of cutting back the numbers of IMGs accepted for residency training not only because of the threat that it holds for less care for large numbers of needy patients but because of the financial implications of such a cutback on the future well-being of teaching hospitals in a limited number of states where the training and subsequent employment of IMGs looms large, such as in New York, New Jersey, Michigan, and a limited number of other states. Congress is very disinclined to compound its current problems in the hope of easing its future challenges. To put it simply: the political risks of cutbacks now appear to a majority of the members of Congress to exceed the gains from moderating a prospective but still unproved dysfunctional physician surplus.

Just consider the situation in the New York region, which provides residency training for three to four times more IMGs than its population would justify if IMGs were distributed across the principal states in accordance with their populations. Consider further that despite its very large total expenditures for health care, estimated at $53 billion for 1999 in New York City alone, amounting to 20 percent of the City's gross domestic product (GDP), and with New York State financing Medicaid more liberally than any other large state, New York City still has almost 30 percent of its below-65 population uninsured at this point in time. And consider further that its eleven acute care public hospitals, as well as many under nonprofit sponsorship, are heavily dependent on IMGs for providing health care services to the large low-income populations that comprise many or most of their patients, ambulatory and inpatient. In light of these facts, it is not surprising that Spencer Foreman, CEO of Montefiore Medical Center, testified recently on behalf of the Greater New York Hospital Association advising policymakers in Washington not to act favorably on the advice of the several national medical organizations that have requested it to reduce the number of IMGs to be admitted to the United States in the years ahead.

But even if Congress were not to make any significant changes in the number of IMGs admitted to the United States for residency training in the near, middle-term future it would be a misreading of present facts and likely future trends to assume that the medical school–graduate medical educational structure will remain unaffected by the changes that are likely to occur in the health care sector in the years ahead, up to 2030. One cannot but be surprised by the stability in the U.S. medical school structure since the mid-1980s, particularly in the case of its 125 allopathic medical schools. There was one closure, Oral Roberts University in 1990-91; and one merger of the Medical College of Pennsylvania and Hanemann University in 1995. In the early 1980s (1983-84), the U.S. had 124 allopathic medical schools in operation and at the end of the century (1999-2000) it had the same number in operation, 124.

Despite the striking stability in the number of public and private allopathic medical schools in operation, numbering 124, between 1983 and 1984 and the end of the century, one must not assume that the next three decades will see a comparable stability. Consider the following: the federal government has recently signaled that it plans to reduce by a significant amount its prospective funding for GME. Consider further, the steadily growing number of academic health centers and teaching hospitals that are characterized by a steadily declining patient occupancy. The State of Pennsylvania had to participate in the rescue and reassign responsibility for the Allegheny Medical School when its parent organization went into bankruptcy. Stanford and the University of California (San Francisco) entered into an affiliation with the intention of reducing duplicating functions and excessive expenditures, but the effort failed. Mt. Sinai Medical School and New York University were originally interested in a more comprehensive merger plan that went off track and was implemented only after the future independence of their two medical schools was assured.

As this selective historical review indicates, the complex interactions among policy initiatives by different participants in the physician supply arena have resulted in an odd mosaic, whereby policies that benefit one group often have adverse effects on others. For instance, it is true that expanding the number of physicians has had some benefits in broadening access, but it has also led to much larger expenditures. Therefore, a more inclusive consideration of physician and medical personnel supply issues is required, in which the financing of the system, ease of access, and the modes of delivery are all part of the analysis. Furthermore, absent a comprehensive analysis, it would be impossible to reach agreement about system-wide innovations and changes.

There is no way to outguess at the beginning of the twenty-first century whether the stability in the medical school infrastructure during the first quarter century is likely to parallel that of the past two decades. But it is not difficult to identify some challenges, the early signs of which were already visible in the year 2000. The first involves the growing evidence that most medical schools continue to depend excessively on training based on in-patients while most informed observers have been recommending for some time the desirability of expanding the training of both medical students and residents in ambulatory sites. Admittedly, this is not an easy shift to make and will almost certainly lead to higher prices resulting from more costly supervision in ambulatory environments. But sooner or later, the additional funding will have to be found if the new generation of physicians is to be appropriately prepared to care for more ambulatory patients.

A closely related challenge are the changes that lie ahead as a consequence of the continuing growth in the number of patients with chronic conditions, in large measure the result of more patients living into their seventies, eighties, and even nineties and beyond, with more of them preferring to live at home rather than in nursing homes. While there have been some experiments at a few academic health centers for joint education and training of medical students, nurses, and other clinical support personnel, the efforts have been quite modest. But the odds favor a growing shift in the patient-physician relationship, where in the future the physician will serve as head of a medical team with nurses, other non-physician clinicians, and medical technicians providing considerable routine care, particularly to the homebound, with clearly delineated responsibilities within their respective areas of competence.

The steady increase in the need and demand of a growing elderly population for a larger range of health care services—preventive, diagnostic, procedural, rehabilitative, and still others—will increase the pressures on all payers to explore improved structures and operations that hold the promise of contributing to expanded and more effective medical outcomes, while moderating the use of costly resources. There is little, if anything, in the recent experience of the U.S. health care system that suggests that improved outcomes can be achieved at non-accelerating costs. However, the challenge remains to pursue the two goals simultaneously since the American people will sooner or later decide that they are no longer willing to devote a steadily growing share of their national income to improved health care, given the other pressing demands on the nation's restricted resources.

The only prospect of accomplishing the joint goals of better health care at a sustainable cost is to identify examples from other sectors of the economy in which more and better outcomes were achieved without constantly expanding costs. The three principal clues that can be extracted from twentieth-century U.S. experience are the potentials of research, the reorganization of production, and the economizing in the use of high cost talent that might contribute to more desirable outputs at a constrained cost.

Looking at the last third of the twentieth century, that is, since the implementation of Medicare and Medicaid, it is clear that research added considerably to the effectiveness of medical care and the prolongation of human life, but not to the constraint of costs. Further, there is relatively little evidence that the production of improved medical care delivery underwent large-scale change in the last two decades, which contributed to significant gains in outcomes with corresponding moderation of costs. The challenge of improving the system for delivery of additional and more effective medical care to the American people at a sustainable cost remains high on the nation's agenda.

A clue as to how the above challenge might be achieved—and the emphasis is on *might*—is if the health care sector could be reorganized so that its costly personnel, starting with specialist and generalist physicians, could be deployed more effectively than in the past. There is some evidence that such an outcome may be feasible, even if progress to date has been modest.

Over the past decades more and more non-physician clinicians and medical technicians have assumed important roles as members of the medical team. But "the team" is more a concept in formulation than in reality. Most interchanges between patients and the medical care system are with their individual physician. Although the physician, by virtue of education and experience, must remain in charge the opportunities are considerable, some would say great, to expand the scale and scope of the health care team to include nurse practitioners, physician assistants, medical technicians, and others whose greater involvement could contribute to improved outcomes and lower costs. Improved organizational arrangements and improved use of highly educated and costly labor together with improved technology have been the critical factors in the continuing growth of the U.S. economy. There is every reason to look on these same challenges as holding the promise for better health care for the American people at a sustainable cost.

The chapters that follow explore the major challenges associated with the physician supply that hold promise of providing better health care outcomes, within a sustainable and acceptable level of additional total outlays, for Americans during the first three decades of the twenty-first century. Chapters 2, 3, and 4 deal with access, financing, and delivery, respectively, as these relate to physician supply. They explore how changes in the numbers and types of physicians have or have not affected these three main aspects of the system and, at the same time, examine the unsolved problems in these areas that may have an effect on the future of the physician supply. Chapter 5 seeks to identify what the demands on the health care system in 2025-2030 will be in terms of access, financing, and delivery. The demographic challenge in the doubling of the elderly in the two decades between 2010 and 2030 (people getting older and living longer) will be an important aspect in determining the impact of the radical change in the medical personnel that the nation will need. Chapter 6 looks specifically at the potential and trends regarding non-physician clinicians as they relate to the practice of medicine by physicians. Chapter 7 summarizes the findings and the major trends as we see them, discussing the major policy issues as we move forward into the first three decades of the new century. This chapter adopts a pragmatic approach, considering what we can realistically expect to achieve through physician supply policy reform and what not. Finally, chapter 8 explores the overall connections between the U.S. health care system and the issue of physician supply, focusing particularly on how the future of medicine will not be determined solely by the medical profession, which is the continuation of a trend that has been ongoing for the better part of the previous century. The plethora of other interested parties and the changes in demography, as well as in medical technology, and the continuous struggle to ensure quality care at a reasonable cost to the American people all but ensure that the health care arena and the specific area of medical personnel supply will remain, for the foreseeable future, a difficult topic for policymakers.

2

Are More Physicians the Answer?

Access to health care is a multifaceted issue dealing with health insurance, access to physicians, and availability of medical facilities. In this chapter, we concentrate mostly on the second aspect, not because the first and third are unimportant, but because physician supply, the main focus of this volume, relates to access to physicians and more broadly to medical personnel in general. We also comment on selected issues of health insurance and medical facilities as they relate to improved access to health care for Americans.

The interaction between the numbers and types of physicians and other health care professionals and the access that the American people enjoy is extremely complex. Physician supply policies have had at best only marginal effects and compensate for shortfalls in health insurance. No matter how many physicians we have, if a person is uninsured, he/she will end up with poorer access, and fewer interventions. Secondly, physician supply policy has not been very effective in terms of balancing the geographic redistribution of physicians. What the United States has been able to do is alter the numbers, types, and ethnic/racial/gender mix of the physician labor force over the years. What has not been clear, however, are the directions towards which national health planning and policy should move next, given the approximate doubling in the ratio of physicians per 100,000 population during the last third of the twentieth century.

In this chapter we will look more closely at the interactions between efforts to alter the physician supply and to improve access to health care services for Americans. The focus will be primarily on the policy interventions affecting physician supply that had an impact on improving access, leaving for the following two chapters a broadened assessment of how parallel efforts to increase the total financing of the U.S. health care sector and the interactions between the increased personnel supply and much enlarged total health care spending affected the delivery of more and better health care services to most, if not all, of the public.

Policy without Statistics

The federal government began in 1963 to use federal funds, in association with state funding, to increase the number of physicians, a decision that grew out of three related developments that characterized the U.S. health care delivery system after World War II. By the war's end, the era of high-tech medicine had begun. The war had also led to an explosive growth in private health insurance coverage, funded by employers with an attractive federal subsidy, and in the two decades following the war, with the American economy expanding at a rapid rate and the incomes of most groups also advancing briskly, the public sought broadened access to physicians as the key to obtaining expanded access to more and better medical care. The federal government's action was facilitated by the decision of the AMA in 1963 to withdraw its long term lobbying against direct federal funding for medical education in order to concentrate its efforts on defeating the pending Medicare legislation. Congress moved speedily after 1963 to enlarge its initial appropriations to increase the physician supply—as well as the supply of other health care personnel, from nurses to dentists to veterinarians and other non-physician clinicians. After thirteen years, in 1976, Congress concluded that the earlier shortages of physicians had been eliminated or were in the process of being eliminated through the establishment of the forty new allopathic medical schools, together with the expansion in the capacity and enrollments of most of the eighty preexisting medical schools.

In 1960, the United States had about 140 physicians available to care per 100,000 population. By the century's end, the physician supply had increased to just about double the 140 ratio, approximating 280, with most of the expansion reflecting the doubling of graduates from U.S. allopathic medical schools (tables 2.1 and 2.2).

Another factor that led to the increase in the total numbers of physicians, and that played a leading role, especially after the mid-1980s when the U.S. allopathic schools ceased expanding their output of graduates, was the U.S. policy that accepted substantial numbers of graduates of foreign medical schools who entered the United States to pursue their residency training, most of whom remained to practice in the U.S.

Table 2.1
Non-Federal Physicians, Physician to Population Ratios, 1960-1998

	1960	1985	1990	1995	1998
Total Physicians (000)	97	522	584	689	737
Physician to Population Ratio	140	220	237	264	277

Table 2.2
Graduates of U.S. Allopathic Medical Schools, 1960-1999

	1960	1970	1980	1990	1999
Graduates	6900	8900	15600	15400	16100

Table 2.3
Total and 1MG Residents (selected years)

Year	Total	IMG
1985	74,514	12,509
1990	85,330	12,259
1994	97,370	22,721
1996	98,035	24,982
1997	98,076	24,703
1998	98,143	25,531
% change (85-94)	31%	82%
% change (94—98)	1%	12%

Table 2.4
Total and IMG PGY1 Residents (selected years)

Year	Total	1MG
1985	19,168	2,673
1990	18,131	2,689
1994	26,033	7,382
1996	24,170	6,233
1997	24,608	6,105
1998	25,531	6,257
% change (85—94)	36%	176%
% change (94—98)	—6%	—15%

Two further notations about the U.S. physician supply: In earlier decades a considerable number of U.S. citizens went abroad to attend medical school, and after obtaining their M.D. degrees returned to the United States for their residency training before entering practice (table 2.5).

The other source of additional U.S. physician personnel reflects the expansion in the number of osteopathic medical schools and the number of their graduates, together with an ever closer alignment between the graduates of the two sectors with a growing proportion of graduates of osteopathic medical schools entering allopathic residency training programs and later practicing in close association with their allopathic colleagues. But one should not equate the increase in total numbers of physicians with adequate access of health care for the entire population. Both the total numbers, but more importantly the numbers of physicians per 100,000 population, continue to vary substantially among states, with the poorer states like Mississippi having as few as half or even fewer the number of physicians per 100,000 as New York or Massachusetts. This has been a persistent problem these last thirty years, even though the total number of physicians almost doubled following the 1963 legislation. Table 2.6 indicates the divergence in these numbers.

Table 2.5
1MG Residents by Citizenship

Year	U.S. Citizens	Foreign
88	4329	7227
89	4595	8726
90	5067	10949
91	5258	12881
92	5272	15621
93	5162	18558
94	4481	21199
95	4198	22565
96	4205	20462
97	4185	20218
98	4266	20685

Table 2.6
U.S. Physicians (in thousands) (totals and per 100,000 ratios), Selected States

Physicians

State	1980	1990	1995	1998
Total	468	616	720	739.5
California	68.5	78.2	86.3	88
Connecticut	9.3	10.7	12.1	12.3
Florida	26.5	31.4	37.9	40
Massachusetts	19	21.4	25.4	26.2
Mississippi	3	3.7	4.1	4.6
Nevada	1.5	1.9	2.7	3.1
New Jersey	18	20,5	23.9	24.6
New York	56.1	60.7	70.7	72.8
Ohio	20.8	23.2	26.9	27.5
Texas	27.9	31.6	38.3	41.2

Ratio per 100,000

Physicians

State	1980	1990	1995	1998
Total	200	237	264	270
California	265	272	275	277
Connecticut	302	332	372	375
Florida	235	251	269	278
Massachusetts	330	364	420	428
Mississippi	124	144	155	165
Nevada	172	175	178	185
New Jersey	242	267	302	308
New York	318	339	391	397
Ohio	197	213	242	248
Texas	172	188	206	210

In 1964, Congress passed a much-expanded Civil Rights Act on which it had failed to act during the preceding year because of President Kennedy's assassination. The act's initial emphasis had been aimed at removing racial prejudices in admitting African Americans to U.S. medical schools, but during the redrafting of the Civil Rights Act of 1964 the sponsors also prohibited discrimination based on gender. As a consequence, the future mix of physicians in the United States changed markedly. The number of African Americans admitted to and graduating from U.S. medical schools increased four-fold, from 2 to 8 percent, but the more striking change over the next decades was the major expansion in the numbers and proportion of women who entered the practice of medicine. At the time that the Civil Rights Act was enacted, the United States had the lowest percentage of women physicians, around 8 percent, of any advanced nation. By century's end women accounted for 43 percent of the newly enrolled freshman class in U.S. medical schools. The following quote from a 1995 COGME report on Women in Medicine is indicative:

> The goal is…to increase physician's understanding of the unique aspects of women's health in order to improve health care delivery…. Since change begins with a vision, a new paradigm in women's health is presented. It is based on broad principles recognizing the gender sensitive biological mechanisms and psychosocial factors that influence health and disease characteristics and patterns….

From 1965 to 1999, the percentage of United States Medical Graduates (USMGs) that are female rose from 6.9 percent to 43 percent. That rise is also reflected in the rising percentage of female physicians in active practice. Their percentage has increased from 7 percent in 1970 to 21 percent in 1999. It is estimated that by 2010, 30 percent of all practicing physicians will be females.

One must quickly add that even after the passage of a third of a century, women practice fewer hours per year than their male colleagues; a much larger percentage of women than men practice as generalists; and women are underrepresented among senior faculty members of medical schools. Furthermore, women still make less money than men even when one controls for specialty and age. On average, they make $5,000 to $15,000 less for physicians under forty years old, $15,000 to $30,000 less for ages 40-49, and $5,000 to $50,000 less for age fifty and above, depending on the specialty. Despite these several differences, the practice of medicine, which had been an overwhelmingly male profession in the early 1960s, had been transformed into an almost equal number of men and women physicians entering the profession at century's end.

Women in medicine are expected to be more sensitive to women's issues and also more likely to follow a generalist career. This holds true for women graduating from both allopathic and osteopathic schools. More than half of all women physicians enter general and family practice, pediatrics, obstetrics-gynecology, psychiatry, and internal medicine much more frequently than other specialties. This is true for 60 percent of allopathic female doctors and 71 percent of osteopathic female doctors who select careers in these specialties. And this is one additional reason why their differentially greater increase in relation to males has been especially welcomed.

As table 2.8 shows and as has been pointed out earlier, the numbers of women that apply, get accepted, enroll, and graduate from medical school have increased tremendously and they account today for more than 45 percent of current graduates.

In 1965, Congress took two further actions, the first to pass Medicare and Medicaid, which, as the next chapter outlines, quickly in-

Table 2.7
Allopathic Physicians by Gender (in thousands)

	1970 (%)	1980 (%)	1990 (%)	2000 (%)	2010 (%)
Total	331 (100)	468(100)	615(100)	670 (100)	677 (100)
Male	305 (92.3)	413 (88.4)	511 (83.1)	543(81.2)	477 (70.6)
Female	25 (7.7)	54 (11.6)	104 (16.9)	126 (19)	198 (29)

Table 2.8
Women and Medical School [women in thousands
(and women as percent of total)], 1965-2000

	1965	1970	1980	1990	1995	2000
Applicants	1.6 (9)	2.7 (11)	10.6 (29.5)	11.8 (40)	19.8 (42.5)	17.4 (45.2)
Enrolled	2.5 (7.9)	3.8 (9.6)	17.2 (26.5)	24.3 (37.3)	28 (41.9)	28.7 (43.2)
Graduates	0.5 (6.9)	0.8 (9.2)	3.9 (24.9)	5.5 (36)	6.5 (40.9)	6.6 (42)

creased the flow of governmental dollars both for the education of residents and for the treatment of the low-income sick. In turn, the new funding had major impacts on care of the elderly (above 65).

But 1965 saw a second Congressional initiative, this one directed at altering the long in place (since the early 1920s) laws and regulations governing the immigration and naturalization statutes and procedures for immigrants seeking to relocate to the United States. Linked to this legislative reform was a new opportunity for foreign-born and foreign-educated medical graduates to enter the United States for residency training, the majority of whom succeeded in later altering their temporary visa so that they could remain in the United States permanently. At century's end, the International Medical Graduates (IMGs) accounted for about 1:4 physicians in active practice in the United States and as we will see at the conclusion of this chapter, the future policy with respect to IMGs remains a much-debated issue on the medical profession's agenda.

Policy by Learning from Experience

In the late 1960s and early 1970s, Congress faced three new legislative initiatives that aimed to increase the physician supply so as to improve access for the groups identified below. In the latter years of President Lyndon Johnson's administration the federal government made sizable amounts of federal funding available to operate a large number of community health centers located in underserved areas, both low density rural locations and low-income urban areas where residents and workers faced great difficulty in obtaining health care services because of the nonexistence of an adequate medical infrastructure of clinics, hospitals, physicians, and support personnel. The federal legislators recognized that its much more ambitious efforts to expand radically the total supply of the nation's physicians would take much too long and even with the passage of time might not be adequately responsive to fulfilling the unmet medical needs of the most deprived subgroups who had limited access even to emergency medical care.

Congress not only appropriated funding for the construction and operation of a growing number of community health centers, but took the further step of recognizing that it would often be impossible for these newly erected clinics to attract the numbers of physicians to provide care to the growing numbers of patients who would seek care. Accordingly, Congress stipulated that nurse practitioners could substitute for physicians; and, further, they would be permitted to bill Medicaid and Medicare directly for the medical care that they provided. Had it not been for the increasing pressures on the federal budget resulting from the prolongation of the war in Vietnam as well as the steeply increasing rate of inflation the number of community health clinics would have continued to increase rapidly.

But the growing tightness of the federal budget did not stop Congress from passing the National Health Service Corps (NHSC) in 1970, which reflected a growing awareness on the part of the legislators that despite the proposed doubling of the physician supply it could not be relied upon to resolve the serious shortfalls in the number of practicing physicians in a large number of underserved areas, primarily rural and low-income urban neighborhoods. The NHSC was established under the Emergency Health Personnel Act of 1970 as a program of the U.S. Public Health Service. Until 1980, providers were federal employees. Today, however, very few providers receive pay and benefits directly from Washington. Instead they are employed by the community health center or other local provider for whom they work. Direct federal assistance takes the form of scholarships or loan repayments. This part of the program was established in 1972 and amended in 1987. The NHSC made federal incentives available for physicians and other health professionals who were willing to relocate for a specified number of years to practice in an "underserved area" in the hope that many would remain once their initial obligation had been fulfilled.

The NHSC expanded steadily during the 1970s, and by the early 1980s the number of physicians serving in the Corps numbered around 2,200. Over the years, more than 18,000 providers have served in the NHSC. In the early 1980s, the newly elected Reagan administration, seeking ways to constrain Congressional outlays, reviewed the program and found sufficient weaknesses and malfunctioning that it all but cannibalized the program which was later renewed under Bush and Clinton but never returned to its pre-1980 scale.

In 1971, Congress recognized that even with its earlier actions that had led to the establishment of a large number of community health centers and subsequently to the establishment of the NHSC, more had to be done to speed the redistribution of physicians into shortage areas. With coaching from the medical leadership in the less populous mid-western states, such as Kansas and Missouri, as well as in several other states, Congress decided in 1971 to fund newly established family practice residencies on the assumption that some or many of the graduates of such programs, having become acquainted with the local and regional population and its health care needs, would elect, after the completion of their residency, to practice in these areas. The Congressional initiative was well received by many of the academic health centers located in smaller communities, and by the beginning of the 1990s family practice residencies could boast the third largest number of residents in training, after internal medicine and general surgery. Between the beginning and the end of the 1990s, assisted by the expanded enrollments into managed care plans and the heavy reliance of these plans on generalists for gatekeepers, many of the research-oriented academic health centers that had earlier turned their backs on starting family practice residencies began to reconsider. By the late 1990s, family practice residencies had achieved the largest gain of any residency program, from just under 7,000 to 10,700.

Policy Shaped by Statistics

After sustained and expanded efforts to increase the physician supply, Congress passed legislation in 1976 proclaiming that the prior serious shortage of physicians had been eliminated through the long-sustained federal support for the expansion of both the number of U.S. medical schools in operation, together with a much enlarged number of medical school graduates that would be graduating in the near future, which would result in a doubling of the annual output from around 8,000 in the late 1960s to 16,000 by the early 1980s.

In declaring the physician shortage at an end, Congress added a gratuitous threat to the effect that it would no longer make any type of medical training funds available in the future unless the applicant medical school could demonstrate that at least 50 percent of its graduating class had selected a generalist residency program. A few medical schools entered a strong protest, pointing out that this new provision was inappropriate both because Congress should not seek to regulate the residency choices that medical school graduates make; and further because medical schools were in no position to influence, much less assure, that their graduates would meet the new Congressional objective. A few years later Congress rescinded the objectionable requirement.

The more important action that the Congress took when it declared the physician shortage problem to have been solved by (a)
the liberal funding program of thirteen years that had resulted in an
increase of about 50 percent in the number of allopathic medical
schools; (b) the expansion of most of the existing medical schools;
and (c) the prospective doubling in the number of annual graduates
from around 8,000 in the late 1960s to double that figure, a few
years ahead, by the early 1980s, was its decision to assess and moni-
tor the future physician supply. Uneasy that its strenuous efforts to
eliminate the earlier shortage of physicians might lead to a prospective surplus Congress established the Graduate Medical Education
National Advisory Committee (GMENAC) to undertake an in-depth
study of the physician supply issue in the near and middle-term future. In 1980, GMENAC reported that it estimated that the United
States would face a surplus of about 70,000 physicians in 1990
(536,000 available/466, 000 required) and somewhat over-double
supplies (145,000) by the century's end. The GMENAC report was
the first time that the IMG issue had been identified as one of broad
concern. In the Committee's words: "the expected entry into practice over the next ten years of 40,000 to 50,000 graduates of foreign
medical schools accounts for more than half of the 70,000 physician surplus." GMENAC also predicted the increase in the number
of non-physician clinicians, raised questions about the uncertainties
entailed in predicting future costs of medical education; and in assessing the role of medical schools in specialty choice and a number
of other related issues.

Although GMENAC had a good staff and had consulted widely
during its four-year investigation its conclusions and recommendations released at the beginning of the 1980s attracted little attention
and still less support. There was relatively little if any substantiation
in the experience of either generalists or specialists that pointed to
early signs that a serious surplus of physicians was only a few years
off. Most practicing physicians were as busy as they wanted to be
and their earnings were still heading up. True, one could point to a
few locations, particularly on the West Coast and more particularly
in Southern California, where a minority of physicians, mostly specialists and subspecialists were not as busy as they wanted to be, but
their situation was more or less unique.

But the mid-1980s saw the beginning of changes in the open-
ended financing of the U.S. health care system that followed upon

the implementation of Medicare and Medicaid in 1966, which had resulted in close to a six-fold increase in current dollars in national health expenditures (NHE) between 1965 and 1980, from $41 billion to just under $250 billion! By 1983, Congress had decided that it was time to alter its payment system for hospital care for Medicare patients from cost-plus (an allowance for capital outlays) to a prospective payment system to be guided by average reimbursement outlays based on "diagnostic related groups" (DRGs)

As we will see later on, a related development was the steady decline in the previous, long, upward trend in the use of acute care hospitals, an outcome of both the severe recession that led many patients to delay their hospitalization for elective procedures; and the further fact that advances in medical technology enabled acute care hospitals to shift many critical treatments from in-patient to ambulatory (same day) procedures. Although the severe recession was brought under control by late 1982, the prior level of admissions and length of stays in acute care hospitals were permanently lowered by as much as 20 percent, if not more.

Policy Based on Power

The third long-time change, dating from the early to mid-1980s, again with Southern California in the lead, saw corporate employer-managed care plan informal alliances aimed at curtailing the steep annual increases in the health insurance coverage rates that the employer groups had to meet in order to provide coverage to their employees. The interactions between the growth of managed care plan enrollments and the broader issues of the physician supply took the better part of a decade—until the early mid-1990s—to reach a point where the consequences of the exploding growth of managed care enrollments commanded the attention of growing numbers of patients, physicians, as well as both state legislatures and Congress. The managed care companies decided that the preferred way to controlling the costs of enrolled patients was to require them to consult their gatekeeper generalist physician before accessing any high cost medical intervention such as consulting specialists and undergoing expensive diagnostic procedures; or being authorized to seek hospital admission; or extend their hospital stay beyond what their plan considered necessary.

The rapid growth of managed care companies in the 1980s and early 1990s focused attention on one aspect of physician supply that had surfaced as early as the beginning of the 1970s but had failed to gain broad national attention. As noted above, the managed care revolution created an additional demand for generalist physicians who would act as gatekeepers, overseeing the medical needs of the rapidly growing numbers of managed care patients with an aim of moderating their steeply rising expenditures. The fact that selected physician specialist groups were also facing a smaller or greater decline in the demand for their services brought the specialist-generalist question to the fore. After a 2:1 ratio of specialists to generalists during the years following the initiation of Medicare and Medicaid, the number and proportion of generalists increased strikingly by the mid-1990s only to see the ratio reverse once again as the century came to an end (table 2.9)

Part of the recent reversal may be the consequence of increasing numbers of managed care companies responding to the growing complaints of many enrollees to permit them to visit their specialists without prior consultation with their gatekeeper physician. What was frequently overlooked in the recent debates about the appropriate ratio of generalists to specialists was the earlier finding of Dean Menderhall and his associates that many specialists serve as the principal physician to patients with chronic diseases.

By the late 1980s-early 1990s, managed care companies found themselves under growing attack, having to answer more and more

Table 2.9
**Percentages of Primary Care and Non-Primary Care Physicians (selected years
1960-1998)**

Year	Primary Care	Non-Primary Care
1960	53	47
1965	45	55
1970	38	62
1981	34	66
1988	33	67
1995	40	60
1996	39	61
1998	34	66

questions about their practices. Patients or the relatives of patients whose conditions had worsened or who had died because of the unwillingness of their managed care plan to approve one or another costly procedure began to sue, and occasionally to be awarded large damages. Further, a large number of patients with chronic illnesses who were being cared for by a specialist physician complained about having to receive new clearance from their gatekeeper before they could visit their specialist.

Slowly but surely, more and more physicians in active practice became increasingly hostile to following the arbitrary actions of managed care plans, which often included their being dropped from the plan's rolls, having their treatment recommendations denied, and suffering a host of other "interferences" by a managed care company's bureaucrats canceling or modifying proposed treatments that they had recommended for their patients.

By the late 1990s, an increasing number of state legislatures were being pressured by disgruntled enrollees, physicians, and hospitals to restrict the earlier freedom of managed care companies to interfere with the long-established autonomy of the physician to determine his or her patient's treatment plan. At a minimum, the petitioning groups sought legislative approval to sue the managed care plans in the event of adverse consequences to those that amended or cancelled the patient's physician plan of treatment.

As the new century was ushered in, the managed care industry came under increasingly severe pressures in the health marketplace, in the stock market, in the political arena, and in the courts, with at least two early impacts on the physician supply. While the growing reliance of the managed care industry on "gatekeepers" had led to a rapid increase in the number of residents pursuing a family practice residency, the backlash of the last few years, particularly from patients, resulted in a subsequent reduction by managed care plans in requiring patients with chronic diseases to seek prior approval for visits to specialists.

A further evidence of the disenchantment of growing numbers of enrollees with managed care plans has been the shift from an HMO type of coverage to POS or PPO types of coverage where the enrollee has more freedom of choice in the selection of his or her physician, usually based on the payment of an additional fee. Although the full extent to which federal and state governments will alter, through legislation and administrative actions, the power relations that had dominated the U.S. health care marketplace during the first half of 1999 must still await the passage of additional time; the odds are strong that for-profit managed care companies will see their power to determine unilaterally physician–patient relations, already considerably eroded, still further eroded in the early years of the new century. This is not to say that the evolving health care sector will turn its back on seeking to moderate the rate of annual increases in NHE but only that the managerial staffs of managed care companies will no longer be in a position to alter unilaterally the prior arrangements that the patient in consultation with his physician has decided upon. The American voter never planned and never agreed to for-profit managed care companies shifting decision-making power from physicians to themselves. By 2002, it is clear that a reverse power shift is underway once more strengthening the decision-making role of the physician.

Policy to Control the Physician Supply

Congress recognized shortly after the early implementation of its major effort to increase by an order of magnitude the number of physicians per 100,000 that it could not stand by and do nothing to help moderate the inadequate number of physicians available to the rural population, particularly to those who lived far distant from any urban concentration. As was noted earlier, Congress acted to increase the number of physicians willing to locate in rural areas by establishing community health centers in the late 1960s, the NHSC in 1970, and federal funding for family practice residencies in 1971. The Tenth Report of the Council of Graduate Medical Education (COGME) released in February 1998, dealing with "Physician Distribution and Health Care Challenges in Rural and Inner-City Areas," noted that in the smallest rural cities, those with between 2,500 and 10,000, not located near a large city or suburb and with a ratio of as few as 53 physicians per 100,000 population, some proportion of the 50 million people living in these rural areas were unable to access any of the 9 percent of the nation's physicians who practice in such areas. Just consider that in the large metropolitan centers, those with more than 1 million population, the ratio of physicians per 100,000 population exceeded 300 in the mid-1990s in contrast to the 53 practicing in the smallest rural areas.

But the above cited report makes the point (p. 22) that extreme poverty, a lack of physical and cultural amenities, and a predominance of ethnic minority populations create barriers to attracting the minimum number of physicians required to care for them. The report goes on to point out that medical school graduates of rural origin, residents who were exposed during some or all of their training period to practicing among a rural population, as well as physicians who select a family practice residency, are more likely to establish a rural practice (p. 23) While each of these efforts helped, as well as selected other efforts under the initiative of the states and of the private sector, such as the Area Health Educational Centers (AHECs), most rural areas failed to attract even the minimum numbers required.

The more complicated aspects of the physician supply question relate to metropolitan settings, which it must be recalled are home to more than four out of every five residents in the United States. And as noted earlier the largest metropolitan areas with more than 1 million population have over 300 physicians per 100,000 population, with small metros, below 1 million, having 235 physicians per 100,000. Among the important characteristics of urban areas that bear directly on the issues of access to physicians are the following: the relatively small numbers of generalists in private practice who have been willing to establish a practice in low-income neighborhoods; the high proportion of the local population that is uninsured and is not on Medicaid; the frequently low reimbursement rate that the states have established for routine office visits for persons on Medicaid; and the additional shortfall in the number of underrepresented physicians from minority groups to match the large numbers of the local population that belong to an underrepresented minority. In 1994, the senior author of this manuscript pointed out in an article in *JAMA* 271, 464-467, that in the nation's four largest metropolitan areas, the lowest-income neighborhoods had ratios as low as 1 provider in private practice per 10,000 population in contrast to high-income neighborhoods which boasted of 1 physician in private practice to 300 population. The differential access between wealthier and poorer urban districts, even within the same city, is best illustrated by the case of New York City, as table 2.10 indicates.

The startling and disturbing figures of table 2.10 indicate why the urban poor in the nation's largest cities have long relied on public and nonprofit neighborhood clinics—and even more on the care of the emergency rooms and clinics of neighboring hospitals, especially public hospitals that see themselves and are seen by others as "safety-net institutions"—as the principal providers of basic care to

Table 2.10
Patient Care Physicians by Practice Setting, per 100,000
Population in the NYC Region, 1994-1999

	1994			1999		
	office-based	hospital-based	total	office-based	hospital based	total
Region						
Bronx	100	112	212	118	105	223
Kings	110	108	218	142	107	248
Manhattan	501	390	891	560	369	929
Queens	130	106	236	160	100	260

the local low-income population. In selected metropolitan centers such safety-net institutions rely to a marked degree on residents in training, many with IMG status, to provide much of the medical care, usually in association with nurse practitioners and physician assistants.

The heavy reliance of the local poor in urban centers on the hospital emergency rooms and clinics that are able and willing to care for patients who lack insurance coverage and cannot pay out of pocket has at least two correlates. Many patients delay seeking care up to a point where their conditions have worsened and instead of being able to be treated as ambulatory patients they frequently have to be admitted as inpatients because their asthma requires multi-day attention, as is also the case when their severe colds has developed into influenza or pneumonia. And the correlative shortcoming that many/most of the uninsured low- income group faces is that they generally fail to see the same physician on return visits, which, in turn, deprives them of much helpful professional advice and guidance. The shortfall in the number of physicians willing to practice in low-income areas and particularly among low-income minority groups is dually difficult to alter in a society and culture such as prevails in the United States where individuals are free to choose where they prefer to live and work, the only exceptions being in times of national mobilization or war. Although an occasional leader of American medicine has recommended national legislation requiring physicians who complete their residency to work for two or more years in a designated shortage area, the proposal never gained much attention or support. Further, while the physician to population ratio tended to be lowest in low-income rural areas, with more and more of the total U.S. population resident in metropolitan areas (over 80 percent in recent years), the access problem increasingly reflects the disinclination of most physicians in metropolitan areas to establish or maintain practices among the uninsured and the poor, since their earnings and working conditions would be much inferior than if they practiced among middle- and upper-income groups in other areas of the city or in the suburbs.

To address the issue of uneven access in low-income urban areas, mostly populated by minorities, the AAMC launched, in 1991, a project called 3000 by 2000. Since minorities were underrepresented in U.S. admissions to medical schools, the project's goal was to in-crease the number of minority students that entered medical school each year in order to reach 3,000 by the year 2000. As of mid-2000, the results of the program were mixed at best. As table 2.11 indi-cates, prior to the start of the program the percentage of matriculants from minority groups had increased significantly between the late 1960s and mid-1970s, when it stood at 10 percent. In 1990, this percentage was for all intents and purposes the same. Since Project 3000 by 2000 began, the number increased until 1996. At that point, there was no further increase in the number of minority matricu-lants; in fact a decline occurred. The end result was that as of the year 2000, the total number of first-year minority enrollment was 2,088.

Whereas the project appeared in the first few years to be working well, the second half of the program failed to meet its target. Never-

Table 2.11
African Americans and Hispanics and Medical School,
1970-2000

	1970	1980	1990	1995	2000
African American Applicants	1250	3268	3062	5154	4184
Enrolled	808	1548	1744	2340	2088
Graduates	——	1086	1326	1625	1900

theless, the point must be made that the project indicates that the AAMC has been sensitive to the issue of minority representation and will probably continue to be so.

Policy Challenges: A Physician Surplus Ahead

In 1993 and 1994, two major studies were undertaken by leading members of the academic medical community, Jonathan Wiener of Johns Hopkins University and David Kindig of the University of Wisconsin, each of whom concluded that the United States faced a serious surplus of physicians, more particularly, physicians who were in specialty or subspecialty practice.

Their estimates of the number of "surplus physicians" are of the order of 150,000. Each found that the number of primary care physicians was more or less balanced with what the market needed and wanted. There is no question that the professional reputation of the authors, and the prestigious journals that published their articles, affirmed or reaffirmed the consensus of organized medicine that the country had already entered a condition of a physician surplus or would soon confront such a surplus. The Institute of Medicine that addressed the issue of the physician supply in 1997 was unable to reach a unanimous decision as to whether or not the country was already confronted with an excess supply, but the burden of its analysis and conclusion left little question that the United States would soon be entering a world of surplus, if it had not already entered it.

In the latter half of the 1990s, the earlier concern with the current and/or prospective surplus in the physician supply oddly enough fell off the national health policy agenda. Even though the earnings of physicians declined in 1994 for the first time since the nation emerged from the severe recession of the early 1980s, they quickly bounced back in 1995. Admittedly, in the late 1990s, some residents who were completing their training did not find the type of practice opportunity that they had anticipated when they first entered their residency training, but almost all of them were able to enter practice even if not in their preferred location or preferred specialty. There were no reports of recently licensed physicians having to find a temporary job in the post office or driving a cab as had been the case in the depressed 1930s.

Although the Council on Graduate Medical Education (COGME) that had been established in 1986 to advise Congress and the federal government about the future supply and demand for residency training had recommended early on that Congress reduce the number of foreign-born International Medical Graduates admitted for residency training to the United States to no more than 10 percent of the number of U.S. graduates, instead of the 30 percent that prevailed during most of the 1990s, Congress has decided, at least up to the end of the century, not to act on this advice. In 1997, a number of concerned medical professional groups—the Association of American Medical Colleges, the American Medical Association, the Association of Colleges of Osteopathic Medicine, the American Osteopathic Association, the Association of Academic Health Centers, and the National Medical Association—joined together to petition Congress to cut back the number of foreign-born IMGs to the earlier recommended 10 percent of U.S. medical school graduates.

But Congress has not been persuaded and as of 2002 has taken no major action to follow this conjoint recommendation. Clearly, Congress has not been overly concerned that the United States currently or even prospectively faces a significant overage in physicians. A large number of Congressmen continue to hear from constituents in rural areas and in the urban poverty neighborhoods about the difficulties that poor and uninsured persons continue to face in accessing physicians. They are also cognizant of the fact that in a number of states such as New York, New Jersey, Connecticut, Michigan, and a few others IMGs in residency training provide a considerable amount of the patient care provided by safety-net hospitals and clinics in these states. Further, they know that a considerable number of IMGs when they complete their residency training accept positions in communities that are severely short of physicians and that have encountered great difficulty in attracting graduates of American medical schools. Although many IMGs later relocate, some remain in the shortage areas; and in any case they represent at least an important interim addition to the available physician supply in communities that have difficulty in attracting U.S. physicians.

Finally, Congress is aware that a few of the states, including the hospitals in the New York region, train a disproportionate number of IMGs for which they receive critically important additional federal revenue. The teaching hospitals in the New York region train about 12 percent of IMGs, about four times its population ratio which results in an additional billion dollars or so to the region's annual hospitals' revenue. While there would be some potential gains to many Congressmen if the IMG monies could be more evenly distributed, they apparently appreciate that a major reallocation of training funds for IMGs or for GME more broadly could cause more trouble than it is worth. At least they have not seen fit to act either to reduce significantly the number of IMGs or the allocation of the funding for their training.

As of the early twenty-first century, the issue of access continues to influence all discussions about American health care. As we have seen, physician supply policies by government, the private sector, and the profession have over the years sought to address many aspects of the access issue with varying degrees of success. At the same time, the nation has seen its health care expenditures increase dramatically, a development that has also impacted the demand and the supply for physicians. We now turn our attention to the assessment of how greater funding for the health care sector has impacted the delivery of health care services to the American people.

New funding Streams

3

Financing of Health Care

The issue of the U.S. physician supply cannot be analyzed without understanding the financing of the U.S. health care sector. It is important to emphasize that until the end of World War II and shortly thereafter the United States paid relatively little attention to issues involving the physician supply or the federal financing of health care services. There was relatively little that the best trained physicians could do other than provide comfort care to their patients when they fell ill or were injured and most health care financing was met by out of pocket payments of consumers, philanthropic donations to hospitals, and modest appropriations, largely from local and state governments. Total national health expenditures (NHE) at the end of World War II were around 4 percent of GDP. But that quickly changed.

An internal inconsistency has developed in U.S. health care policy that has led to a number of confounding issues affecting the physician supply. On the one hand, Americans want more and better health care extended, if possible, to all citizens, and on the other hand, they also desire to control total health expenditures. These opposing forces have led to the stand-off in health care financing that we observe today. With continuous new funding streams entering the system, government, nonprofit institutions, and private sector companies have tried to respond to the first challenge by introducing a number of cost control measures. At the same time, each injection of new funds into the system has created new political interests, which seek to protect current payment mechanisms.

This political and institutional environment has created the context in which physician supply issues interact with financing. The American approach towards the financing of its health care system has led to the institutional dominance of the hospital in the nation's health care delivery. It has contributed towards more research, more specialism, and more physicians. It has led to a relative increase in the number of specialists despite the 1980s and early 1990s focus on more generalists. It has led to the concentration of physicians in urban centers and wealthy suburbs where they could better assure themselves of earning a satisfactory or high income and engaging in a satisfying practice. It has also led to the observed loss of physician autonomy in the later 1980s-early 1990s and to the subsequent struggle by them to regain it. Each physician issue has roots that can be traced back to the financing of the U.S. health care system. To answer questions such as the total number of physicians, the location and types of their practices, the numbers of non-physician clinicians, etc., we must first come to terms with the ways in which the United States finances its health care system.

The Passage of Medicare and Medicaid and the Disconnect between Dollars and Services

The years immediately following the end of the Second World War saw several important changes on the health care front, including the following. During the course of the war, private health insurance coverage by employers for their employees had expanded by several orders of magnitude. The Penicillin Age had commenced, setting the stage for the rapid expansion of high-tech medicine. The federal government decided to begin liberal financing of biomedical research, with federal funds heavily directed to the leading universities and their medical school faculties, but with the understanding that the results of such research could be turned into useful products by the for-profit pharmaceutical industry. And the federal government also made funding available for the first time (Hill-Burton) to help smaller and medium-sized communities build or improve their local hospitals so that they could attract/retain the physicians required to treat the local population. And most hospitals continued the prewar practice of overcharging private patients to help defray the residual costs arising from their charity and part–pay arrangements.

With the advantage of an interested hindsight we now know that the passage of Medicare and Medicaid in 1965 was arguably the single most important event in the financing of health care in the United States in the twentieth century. Hence, this chapter will address three interrelated questions. First, why was this far-reaching federal legislation passed in 1965? A second and even more relevant question is, how did the enactment and implementation of the new legislation result in so many unanticipated as well as intended consequences? The third question asks, what were the effects of these intended and unintended consequences on the nation's future physician supply?

To return to the first question: Why were Medicare and Medicaid passed? A paradoxical but valid reply would note that the passage of Medicare was linked to the success of private health insurance in the immediate post-World War II decades.

In 1940, 12 million Americans, just over 9 percent of a total population of 132 million, had private health insurance coverage. In 1950, the respective figures were 77 million and 152 million, or just over 50 percent. By 1965, the year that Medicare and Medicaid were enacted, there were 139 million insured persons in a total population of 194 million, for a coverage rate of over 71 percent. In short, in a quarter century the percentage of the population with health insurance increased eight-fold, from 9 percent to about 72 percent.

By the late 1950s, the public and the politicians became increasingly aware that two groups of citizens were at great financial risk in case of hospitalization: many of the elderly who having retired no longer had private insurance through their employer; and many of the poor and near poor who were not working, or if working were not offered insurance coverage by their employer or could not afford to buy it in the market. Ironically, the greater the number of people who were covered by private health insurance, the more clear the vulnerability of these uninsured two groups. In the late 1950s-early 1960s, the federal government made special funding available to the welfare commissioners of several states to help them cover the costs of caring for the uninsured elderly. But many of the uninsured elderly wanted nothing to do with the state welfare system, having avoided it throughout their lifetimes, which left the issue of providing access for them on the national agenda.

Running for the presidency in 1960, John F. Kennedy proposed a national Medicare statute, but despite his victory, Congress, under AMA pressures, legislated a program (Kerr-Mills) that provided federal funds to the states for restricted means-tested health benefits for the elderly poor. The American Medical Association (AMA) with the support of many in the business community had launched the largest campaign in its history to defeat Medicare in the early 1960s. In 1964, the political landscape was radically altered, however, by President Johnson's smashing victory over Senator Goldwater, which brought liberal Democrats into control of the Congress. Still, the chairman of the House Ways and Means Committee, Wilbur Mills (D-Ark.), refused to release the Medicare bill for a vote until he was persuaded that the new program would bring new federal funds into the South; and further, that the potential desegregation of Southern hospitals would not embarrass his colleagues and himself.

After the passage of the new legislation, President Johnson sought to reassure the much unsettled leadership of the AMA that nothing would change in the relations between patients and their physicians except that the government would pick up the bills. The federal government would in no way interfere with traditional physician-patient relations predicated on fee-for-service, and physicians would be reimbursed according to the CPR formula-fees that were customary, prevailing, and reasonable. To underscore his support for the status quo, the president stated that he would designate regional Blue Cross plans to administer claims and payments for the hospital sector, thereby minimizing the role of the federal bureaucracy.

One of the immediate effects of the new legislation, which included liberal funding for Graduate Medical Education (GME), was the greater degree of financial freedom that it offered the country's teaching hospitals, especially the top twenty-five research-oriented Academic Health Centers (AHCs).

Since teaching hospitals play a leading role in the education and training of tomorrow's physicians, since they are also the sites for most of the federal government's funding for biomedical research, and since they further provide a considerable proportion of the nation's most sophisticated medical services to the most seriously ill and injured patients we need to look more carefully at the changes in their financing that followed upon the passage and implementation of Medicare, with some attention as well to the correlative impact of Medicaid, and towards the outlays for which the federal government contributes almost 60 percent.

In the fifteen years from 1950 to 1965, the total expenditures of all non-federal acute care hospitals increased more than four-fold, from slightly over $2.1 billion to $9.1 billion annually; by 1980, the figure was just short of $77 billion. Even after adjusting for inflation, hospital expenditures more than doubled during this post-Medicare fifteen-year period. The rise to dominance of the acute care hospital in the U.S. health care system was directly linked to its ability to obtain ever larger flows of funds to finance the improvement and expansion of its diagnostic and therapeutic infrastructure and thereby provide ever larger numbers of Americans with quality hospital care.

President Johnson's reassurance to the AMA that the passage of the legislation would not alter in any significant fashion the operation of the U.S. health care system proved to be unrealistic. The president had misread the extent to which the new role of government as a payer for hospital care, primarily Medicare, would alter the flow of funds and consequently would alter the behavior of all those who participated in the delivery of hospital care to the American people, in particular, hospitals, physicians, patients, hospital supply companies, pharmaceutical firms, and support staff.

The ridiculously low estimates by federal actuaries of the probable costs of the new programs ($10 billion by 1990) contributed to the ensuing difficulties. Elmer Staats, the (1965) Comptroller General of the United States, voiced his unease with the conservative forecasts presented to Congress by the federal actuaries. He doubted that the government would come off so cheaply, but few were listening.

Why did the president's conviction that Medicare could work without altering the basics of the financing and delivery of health care prove to be wrong? Part of the explanation is that the president, Congress, and the public failed to realize at the time that the new Medicare financing arrangements went a fair distance to erode the linkage between (hospital) expenditures and dollar constraints, a constraint that had operated in almost all sectors of the U.S. economy including peacetime defense procurement. Consumer spending in the market is limited by the amount of money that consumers have to spend in meeting their multiple needs and desires. In the public domain, legislatures have employed an appropriations process designed to ensure that public outlays are kept under reasonable control. Even during the Cold War when one of the Armed Services requested a new weapons system, the requisition was subjected to elaborate budgetary review, initially in the Armed Services and in the Department of Defense, latterly in the U.S. Office of Management and Budget, and before various committees of the House and Senate. Medicare, on the other hand, loosened most of the financial constraints under which hospitals had earlier operated, a consequence that was not anticipated or foreseen.

By the time Medicare was enacted, third-party reimbursements already accounted for about 71 percent of all hospital revenues. This left the trustees of hospitals facing the task of raising almost 30 percent of the total operating budget and, in addition, to elicit extra philanthropic funds for capital expansion, new technological equipment, and other capital needs.

Like every sector in the U.S. economy—for-profit, nonprofit, or governmental—hospital care in the pre-Medicare era was still very much dollar constrained. However, it was only a few years after the implementation of Medicare that third-party payments covered over 90 percent of most hospital budgets. The new situation sent a powerful message to the field. It told hospitals that the more they spent the more they would be reimbursed. Hospital trustees had no reason not to go along with administrators who wanted to launch new projects; and administrators, in turn, had no reason to refuse the requests of their clinical staffs for costly new equipment. The new doctrine of "spend more, be reimbursed more," became the new motto of hospital management.

Whereas prior to the new legislation, few hospitals were in a position to borrow funds for expansion or improvement, things changed quickly. The financial community was eager to issue hospital bonds, which were made more attractive because of their tax-exempt status by the federal and most state governments. Investors saw considerable merit in tax-free hospital bonds whose accounts receivable were heavily underwritten by Blue Cross, the large commercial insurance companies, and federal and state governments.

To put it simply: before the passage and implementation of Medicare and Medicaid, most hospitals were seriously constrained if not stressed because of their financial position as they sought to cope with their expanding ambitions to train more specialists and subspecialists to speed the development of high-tech medicine; to broaden and deepen their activities in the area of biomedical research; and to be able to admit, treat, and improve the outcome of their constantly increasing numbers of seriously ill and disabled patients who were admitted for inpatient and, latterly, often for same day care.

Before the passage of Medicare, instead of being the beneficiaries of more than $6 billion annually of special funding for graduate medical educational expenditures (GME) covering the direct and indirect costs of providing such training and providing the residents with a minimum annual stipend, hospitals had to admit smaller or larger numbers of "charity patients" in order to carry out their clinical educational duties since private patients were generally not available for teaching. Within a short time after the passage of Medicare, all patients became "teaching patients," which eliminated the special costs that hospitals had previously incurred because of the admission of considerable numbers of charity patients for teaching purposes.

In addition, Medicare had further effects, especially in terms of the increasing sophistication of medical care by its continued contributions to education, research, and patient care. Medicare, and to a lesser extent Medicaid, strengthened the financial underpinnings of these centers of medical leadership. By the late 1960s, the combined contributions of government—federal, state, and local—accounted for about 70 percent of all medical school revenues.

Medicare also contributed to graduate medical education. First, it provided funds to compensate some of the hospital staff responsible for residency training. Second, it enabled the physicians who treated patients who were not admitted by private physicians to bill the government for their care. Third, it covered the direct (and eventually the indirect) costs for the education and training of residents and fellows. Most importantly, though often overlooked, Medicare became a principal reimburser for a large range of hospital expenditures, from an expanded, better paid staff to a pass-through arrangement for capital outlays.

A closely related matter that is often overlooked: The fact that the new Medicare reimbursement system made it possible for teaching hospitals to pay something approaching a living stipend to their residents; and the further fact that medical students did not have to start repaying the loans that the federal government had advanced them during their medical school years until they had completed their residency training encouraged many of them to prolong the latter, occasionally to a point that their total residency training period came to around ten years, plus or minus.

This prolonged period of residency training was increasingly pursued by many medical school graduates once they became broadly aware that the high tech medical system that was increasingly dominating American medicine was providing the best opportunities and

Robert Ebert's WARNING

the largest income prospects for those who stayed the course long enough to become specialists and subspecialists.

In all these ways, Medicare contributed to the nations' AHCs' ability to pursue their high-tech missions and to send messages to prospective physicians that specialty training was something to be desired and pursued. True, as Robert Ebert had pointed out at the time, concentrating on training more and more specialists and subspecialists meant that the academic health centers were creating their own future competitors; the fact is that they continued down this path because many specialists whom they were training were able to start practices in smaller communities and in the suburbs, which previously had not been able to offer tertiary care to their communities. The fact that for the better part of the first two decades after the passage of Medicare, reimbursement for in-patient hospital care was based on cost plus (for capital expenses) made it considerably easier for many less sophisticated hospitals to find the capital to upgrade themselves.

Further, the constant increase in the number of tertiary care hospitals in locations where they had not earlier existed made it much more attractive for the large numbers of newly trained specialists and subspecialists to open a practice in these communities, thereby deflecting, at least for a time, the explosive surplus of specialists had they been forced to compete in the larger metropolitan centers. This took the edge off Ebert's warning—at least for the time being—which has in the interim stretched to a quarter century and is likely to continue for an even longer period, if not indefinitely.

In summary, the fifteen years after the passage of Medicare led to tremendous increases in national health expenditures. In addition to hospitals, all of the parties involved in the financing, delivery, and use of hospital care found the new environment conducive to the pursuit of their high priority goals. Consider the following: The newly covered elderly found much to admire in the Medicare legislation which enabled them to utilize the voluntary hospital system and to be treated by many of the nation's premier physicians.

Another group that benefited from Medicare's flow of dollars was hospital employees—from the highly trained professionals to the unskilled housekeeping staff. Previously, hospitals had been protected by a differentially lower minimum wage. With the ability of most hospitals to recover whatever they spent came pressures on them to increase their salary scales. In New York City, the wages of workers in the lowest rungs increased during the late 1960s-1970s from one-third below the market to one-third above. This upward tilt in wages and salaries covered all occupational groups.

The newly relaxed financial environment also resulted in gains to physicians who worked in hospitals full-time or part-time. The special GME funding allowed hospitals to pay their residents salaries in the $15,000-$20,000 range in 1980, up from the previous paltry average of $3,500 to $6,000 when Medicare was first introduced.

Much larger gains were realized by experienced full-time physicians such as radiologists, pathologists, and others who negotiated greatly increased rates of payment from hospitals. The clinical staff also profited by Medicare since they were offered reasonable rates of reimbursement for all Medicare patients and, although Medicaid paid less than their existing fees, still they were reimbursed, which previously had often not been the case.

Hospital admissions had increased by 10 million between 1950 and 1965, from over 16 to 26 million, driven mostly by the expansion of private insurance. In the next decade and a half, the number of admissions continued to grow by approximately 10 million, but the rate of growth had dropped from 63 percent to 38 percent.

What these figures do not reveal, however, is the striking acceleration in the per diem and per episode costs of hospitalization, reflecting greater reliance on both unskilled and skilled labor as well as on increasingly costly technology. In 1966, the cost of a hospital day amounted to $75, a hospital episode just under $615. In 1980, comparable expenditures were $245 and $1,900, respectively. After adjusting for inflation, these figures became $86 and $667, respectively. Even with this adjustment the increases in hospital care expenditures provide evidence of the much less constrained financing environment in which bills were simply passed on from those who incurred them to those who paid them. Medicare had instituted a disconnect between health care services and health care expenditures, facilitated the elevation of the hospital as the dominant actor in health care delivery; and further advanced specialism in the minds of both physicians and the public.

So much for Medicare and its direct and indirect consequences. We must now turn briefly to Medicaid, in particular to the 1972 amendment that made routine nursing home care reimbursable for those who could meet its financial eligibility criteria. Who were these beneficiaries? First, they were poor persons who could profit from a stay in a nursing home and certainly in the case of those who fell within the stringent Medicaid asset and income ceilings. A second group that may have had to pay out-of-pocket upon initial admission would find after a short period of institutionalization that they had "spent down" sufficiently so that they were henceforth eligible for Medicaid. Finally, a considerable number of middle-class persons recognized ahead of time that they might require care sooner or later and distributed ahead of time most of their assets to family members in order to qualify for Medicaid.

The 1972 Medicaid amendments resulted in an accelerated growth in nursing home capacity and admissions. Not to be overlooked was the contribution of entrepreneurs who realized the implications of the amendments and quickly started to provide the expanded nursing home capacity. Despite recent trends that indicate that most Americans with chronic illness prefer to be cared for at home, the nursing home sector was one more industry that took advantage of the new, open-ended financing system generated by Medicare and Medicaid. The growth of the nursing home industry stimulated the demand for professionals who came to be known as non-physician clinicians (NPCs). We will later explore their role.

Early Attempts for Expenditure Control

Despite President Johnson's commitment that after the implementation of Medicare and Medicaid nothing would change in the financing and delivery of care, other than that the government would pick up the bills, it is clear from the preceding discussion that a great number of changes were occurring. Over the succeeding years these changes attracted the attention and concern of Johnson's successors in the White House, the members of Congress, most state legislatures, all of whom resorted to regulatory devices aimed at slowing hospital expenditures. Belatedly, employers and private health insurance companies that along with government had primary responsibility for meeting the steeply rising bills took notice and instituted reforms.

In 1969, just three years after Medicare and Medicaid had first been implemented, President Nixon warned that if the current rate of health care spending was not controlled, the financing of the health care system might collapse and in the process jeopardize the future of the U.S. economy. As part of the wage and price controls introduced in August 1971, Nixon was able to put his earlier admonitions into effect. Even after he lifted the controls on most of the economy in January 1973, Nixon retained controls on physician and hospital charges for several additional months.

At the same time, Congress became concerned with health care expenditures. In 1972, it passed the Professional Standards Review Organization Act (PSRO), which required states to establish a physician-led mechanism to assess the justification for hospital admissions and length of stay by patients covered by Medicare. Congress recognized that it might be to the advantage of local providers to exploit the federal treasury. A year earlier, the Executive also set norms for Medicare reimbursement that would limit payment on deviant bills. At the same time, the Medicare statute was amended to extend coverage to all patients suffering from end-stage renal disease irrespective of age.

In 1973, Congress also made available federal funding to encourage the expansion of existing HMOs and the establishment of new ones; however, the regulations were so stringent that the legislation had only a marginal effect on speeding the growth of managed care.

The following year, Congress acted yet again to slow the rate of national and federal spending for health care, It passed the National Health Planning and Resources Development Act which required states to establish a process that would assess the areal need for any new large-scale expenditure for beds or equipment. Without a "certificate of need" the costs would not be reimbursed by Medicare. A few states like New York had earlier introduced CON legislation, but most had eschewed the introduction of CONs. The federal initiative led to the establishment of a large number of areal health planning agencies and a substantial rise in the employment of analysts and clerks. However, as it turned out decisions reached in state capitals about CON had more to do with the political muscle of the applicant than with an objective assessment of areal needs. By 1984 when the federal legislation came up for renewal it had few advocates and was permitted to lapse.

Early in his administration, President Carter sought Congressional approval for a federal initiative aimed at slowing the rapidly accelerating increases in hospital costs. The goal was to limit annual hospital cost increases to 3 percent above the general inflation rate, not the almost 9 percent spread of recent years. In addition to seeking the moderation of federal outlays the proposal included parallel limits for all other payers such as Blue Cross and commercial insurance as well as limits on total hospital capital investment. The proposed legislation was estimated to reduce federal expenditures over a five-year period by $20 billion and to save another $30 billion for the private health insurance sector. As expected, the hospital industry and the medical profession launched a major attack on the bill. Representative Dan Rostenkowski of Chicago, the chair of the Ways and Means Subcommittee on Health, challenged the hospital industry to take the initiative to control the rise in hospital costs. The industry accepted by forming the Voluntary Effort (VE), a coalition of providers and payers whose goal was to reduce the annual rise in hospital costs for 1978 and 1979 by 2 percent below the rate of increase in 1977. The VE had partial success in 1978 but little in 1979.

In the spring of 1979, as inflation continued to accelerate, the Carter administration introduced a new cost containment measure that avoided many of the mandatory constraints of the earlier legislative initiatives, as long as hospital cost increases remained within 1 percent of the medical market price index, with an allowance for population increases. The hospital industry did not buy into this proposal and the bill was defeated in the House of Representatives late in 1979. The leadership of the American Hospital Association had convinced the house members that it would lead a successful campaign to obtain voluntary adherence to a ceiling on hospital reimbursement rates, a boast on which history proved they did not deliver. What happened is that hospital expenditures slowed a bit while the debate was underway suggesting that hospitals were able to constrain cost increases voluntarily. As soon as the legislation did not pass, however, hospital expenditures returned to their previous steep rates of increase.

Cost Control Measures and Managed Care

The Reagan staff during the first presidential campaign had flirted with the idea of placing greater reliance on the competitive market to moderate the steeply rising level of health and hospital costs. But once in office Reagan sought to have Congress reduce its future spending on Medicare, an effort on which the Congress refused to cooperate. In its place Congress agreed to a three-year reduction in the federal contributions to Medicaid. But even the Democratic-controlled Congress recognized that it had to do something, even something radical, to alter the cost-plus formula that had governed Medicare reimbursements for hospital care since the implementation of Medicare at the beginning of July 1966. Reagan's administration had thrown its weight behind the elimination of cost-based reimbursement for in-patient care under Medicare in favor of a prospective payment methodology (PPS) that had been developed at Yale University and was being deployed experimentally in New Jersey. The hospitals, for their part, preferred PPS to its predecessor, the Tax Equity and Fiscal Responsibility Act, 1982 (TEFRA), which set rigid prospective limits on their prices. With generalized bipartisan recognition of the urgency of stanching the relentless increase in hospital cost inflation, the U.S. Senate voted in 1983 to shift to PPS after only nominal debate.

Despite the efforts of the federal government to moderate its outlays for Medicare during the latter 1980s, the 1990 figures for Medicare reimbursements for hospital care had risen from $28 to $69 billion; and for physician services from $8 to $40 billion. A closer look at the second half of the decade reveals the conflicting pressures on Congress both to rein in steeply rising federal spending for health care and its concern to respond to the current needs of different constituencies, primarily two—mothers and children eligible for coverage under Medicaid; and reducing the strain on the elderly having to meet a growing number of supplementary costs.

In a series of actions in the latter 1980s, Congress expanded coverage for low-income families with young children in the hope and expectation of raising the standing of the United States among the advanced nations of the world, many of which boasted a much lower rate of infant mortality. And, in 1988, under the prompting of Secretary Bowen of Health and Human Services, the Reagan administration supported the introduction of new Congressional legislation aimed at reducing the burden on most of the Medicare population resulting from a large number of deductions and supplemental payments that many lower-income elderly persons found increasingly burdensome. The only condition that President Reagan stipulated to obtain his support for this new legislation was that the additional costs of the reforms would be borne by the more affluent Medicare recipients.

To the surprise of most observers, a campaign was launched shortly after the passage of the new legislation to rescind it, by the affluent elderly many of whom already had coverage for some or most of these supplemental charges through post-retirement benefits from their employer, or from one or other Medigap policy which they had previously purchased. They emphasized in their campaign to rescind the 1988 legislation that an affluent couple would pay up to $1,300 per year in extra taxes to the federal government without deriving any personal benefits for themselves. In late 1989, with some few but important exceptions such as the provision of joint Medicare-Medicaid coverage for the poorest of the elderly, Congress rescinded most of the 1988 statute.

As we have just analyzed, in the third of a century after the passage of Medicare and Medicaid, the federal government was catapulted from the fourth into the first position as a purchaser of health care services. By 1980, NHE had increased six-fold from $41 billion in 1965 when Medicare and Medicaid were first enacted to just under $250 billion, a result of the accelerating inflation during the 1970s, and the sizable governmental outlays for Medicare and Medicaid which brought the share of governmental spending in NHE from 25 percent in 1965 to 43 percent at the beginning of the 1980s. The early 1980s marked an important turning point in the U.S. health care sector operations. The severe recession of 1981-82 marked the onset of a new trend in inpatient hospital admissions—a sharp and lasting reversal in the previous growth trend. The conventional wisdom is that because of the bad times in the early 1980s many patients who had contemplated having non-urgent procedures delayed their admissions to a hospital. But the more potent explanation for the drop-off in inpatient admissions probably reflected the gains in medical and surgical technology that enabled physicians to treat many more patients in an ambulatory care setting. And technology also enabled hospital staffs to accelerate their treatment and discharge of patients who still required follow-up care with the result that the last two decades have seen a decline of about 20 percent in the number of discharges from short-term hospitals, bringing the occupancy rate of community hospitals down from 85 percent to 65 percent. With governmental spending for health care catapulting from around $10 billion in 1965 to almost $500 billion by century's end it is not surprising that belatedly Washington paid increasing attention to how it might constrain future federal health care spending, surely after the early 1980s, at which point it could no longer avoid the issue. But one must quickly add that each of the other major spenders—private sector employers who provided most workers with private health insurance coverage; state governments, major funders of Medicaid; and the consumer who covered about 20 percent of all health care expenditures with out-of-pocket payments—one and all had to confront and react to the steeply increasing NHE. The long disconnect between expenditures and services was coming to an end. From 1983 on, providers would increasingly have to answer questions about the efficiency of their operations.

The decade and a half between the early 1980s and the second half of the 1990s saw a revolutionary change in private sector financing of health care services largely as a consequence of corporate employer groups pressuring the managed care companies, the majority operating under for-profit auspices to moderate the double-digit annual increases in their premium rates to cover the costs of providing their employees with health insurance coverage.

By the early 1970s, many large employers had had three decades of experience in providing health care benefits for their employees and the majority of larger and medium-sized firms had been offering such benefits for at least two decades. By and large, they secured group coverage from either a commercial insurance company or from a Blue Cross plan whose price was predicated on the prior experience of the firm in using hospital and physician services. Since the cost of private health insurance was not a large part of total employee costs until the 1980s, most companies were not concerned with the acceleration in their health care benefit costs, particularly if they believed that the benefits were largely a trade-off for higher wages.

In the mid-to-latter 1970s, a few of the more enterprising companies realized that they could adopt a less accommodating posture when negotiating a further improvement in coverage with their employees and decided to explore whether they could achieve any significant savings by assuming all or most of the risks and administrative costs for which they had long paid an insurer. Recognizing that they could safely assume the risks, in whole or in part, the larger companies began to move expeditiously to self-insure since it made little sense to transfer at the beginning of the year to the insurer the capital that would be paid out only over the next twelve months or even longer. This trend was encouraged by the passage of the federal Employee Retirement Income Security Act (ERISA) of 1974, which exempted such plans from state insurance regulation. By 1980, about 36 percent of all employees covered by employer benefit plans

were in self-insured company plans. Beyond this critically important initiative, the employer community saw no easy way for it to
moderate the steep rise in health and hospital costs, which caused its
steeply rising benefit premiums.

By the early 1980s, and in selective markets, that impasse began
to change. Corporate executives, especially in Southern California,
long home to HMOs, encouraged many managed care companies in
their area to seek better rates from local hospitals with a growing
proportion of empty beds and from local physicians with some free
time on their schedules in return for directing more patients to each.
The physicians agreed to act as gatekeepers for the newly referred
patients, an effort that often led to lower total expenditures by controlling the rights of patients to obtain costly outpatient or in-patient
services that his or her physician had recommended without any
control being exercised by the managed care plan.

As these new arrangements spread from Southern California and
selected other locations enabling managed care plans to achieve a
strong market position, the next step was for the employer community to persuade or force their employees to shift from a fee-for-
service type of coverage to a prepayment arrangement, often to an
HMO model. In the decade and a half between the beginning of the
1980s and the mid-1990s, the large majority of the employed population that had traditionally been enrolled in a fee-for-service mode
of private health insurance, was moved over to a prepaid version of
coverage, of which HMOs were a leading model.

The mid-1990s appeared to mark the success of the new managed care model for private health insurance coverage characterized by modest annual increases in premium rates. But each new
year brought new evidence to the fore that the earlier optimism about
the potential of managed care companies to reform the economics
of the U.S. health care sector by controlling the rate of expenditures
while meeting the needs and desires of the insured public was more
a short-term mirage, not a long-term reality. A brief recapitulation of
the countervailing forces that made their presence felt: government
and the courts became more active partners in adjudicating disputes
between patients and their managed care companies; corporate employers discovered that much as they had appreciated the early success of managed care companies to moderate their premium payments, annual renewal rates were once again heading up and their
employees were pressuring them for broader choices, even if they

had to make some contribution to obtaining them. And the physician community that had been caught unaware and unprepared for its loss of power and prestige had begun to recoup some, even much of their lost power.

As of the year 2002, the resolution of these growing tensions between the managed care companies and patients, physicians, and other providers had not yet been resolved but the directions of radical change were increasingly clear. The profitability of many managed care companies has declined markedly; the gatekeeper approach has come under increasing criticism; consumers want more choice of physicians and specialists and many are able and willing to pay extra to obtain it; the physician community is increasingly exercised by the fact that the managed care companies deflect for their own purposes—salaries, administration, marketing—about 15 percent of all health care revenues that they receive, much more than the value of the services that they provide.

But a serious dilemma remains unanswered. If for-profit managed care is not efficient, effective, or economical, what is to take its place? With NHB estimated to exceed $2 trillion annually by 2008 it would make little or no sense to say that the decision-making power should be returned to the consumer and his or her physician even if both are correct in their claim that physicians should recapture much of their lost decision-making. Decision-making power is likely to slip increasingly from the control of the managed care companies, but it is far from clear in the early twenty-first century as to how an improved balance will be achieved among funders, patients, and physicians.

The third principal source of funding of the U.S. health care system in the post-Medicare era has been the out-of-pocket payments made by consumers which, it needs to be recalled, accounted for half of all payments in 1965 when Medicare and Medicaid were first enacted. At the turn of the century, out-of-pocket payments by consumers had declined from around 50 percent to the 20 percent of NHE, or slightly less.

Clearly, the contradictory movements of the steeply declining role for out-of-pocket payments when placed alongside the increasing numbers of the population below 65 who lack any type of health insurance coverage (42 million) or have restricted coverage (30 million) are warnings of more trouble ahead.

This brings us to the fourth of the major funders of the health care system—state (and local) governments—that are estimated by federal officials to account for about 12.5 percent of the near $1.3 trillion of total NHE for the year 2000. Something over 40 percent of all state and local health care outlays are accounted for by payments for Medicaid. During the past decade, more and more of the states, first those with smaller populations, but more recently the large states as well, have put Medicaid managed care plans in place in the hope and expectation that they might assist the states in moderating the steady increases in medical expenditures that they had been encountering. Because a great number of Medicaid beneficiaries were removed from the rolls as a result of the new federal welfare legislation passed in 1996, and further because of the strong labor market in the closing years of the twentieth century, it is difficult to reach firm conclusions about the role that managed care has played in moderating Medicaid payments in relation to the significant changes in the eligibility requirements and the number of enrollees. While the state legislatures that moved aggressively to expand Medicaid managed care did so in the hope and expectation that it would moderate their health care outlays they also looked to some improvements in the quality of care that managed care plans would be able to provide to their enrollees. The fact that some of the largest private sector managed care companies have failed to bid in states that were introducing or expanding managed care coverage for their Medicaid population; and that some of them have actually withdrawn from markets where they had earlier enrolled Medicaid eligibles suggests that it is probably premature to undertake an evaluation in 2002 of the effectiveness of Medicaid managed care plans, especially in the most populous states.

Another related action by state governments has to do with their push for more generalists. In the past few years, eleven states have directed medical schools to focus on the production of more primary care doctors. The laws that were passed, however, were not very strict and contained a number of loopholes. They do, however, hold significance in the sense that state governments have signaled their desire for more primary care physicians. Whether or not their pressures will actually have the desired effect remains to be seen.

As this review has revealed, the passage of Medicare, and to a lesser degree Medicaid, assured large numbers of elderly and disabled workers who had lost their ready access to mainline medical care when they retired would again be able to access both mainline physician and hospital care. But Medicare through its explicit funding for graduate medical education (GME) also greatly accelerated the earlier trend toward more specialist and subspecialist training on the part of new entrants into the medical profession. It further greatly improved the financial position of the nation's leading academic health centers by providing them with a growing pool of well-trained residents to help care for their growing number of more severely ill hospitalized patients; and to assist in their much enlarged research programs. Further, Medicare and Medicaid enabled large teaching and other hospitals to improve their financial position by converting their earlier considerable number of no-pay and part-pay patients into full-pay patients. And because of their much improved financial position the leading academic health centers were able to focus increasingly on their agenda of advancing high-tech medicine via expanded activities in education, research, and hospital care. In doing so, the hospital-physician sectors contributed greatly to the double-digit increases in national health care expenditures and to elevating the federal government into the single largest payer for medical care. And it also provided the political impetus for cost control, which has, in fact, left its mark on both the public and the private sectors.

But when one looks more closely at the efforts of the federal government to moderate the rate of its future expenditures for Medicare as well as the attempts by other payers to moderate their expenditures, the growing non-fit between the citizenry's desire for more and better care and the several payers seeking to constrain their payments becomes clear. As of the start of the twenty-first century, this is what one can report. The Bipartisan Commission established to come forward with recommendations for the long-term reform of Medicare was unable to agree on an acceptable proposal. The presidentially sponsored Patients Rights Bill is not moving. The drug benefits for Medicare beneficiaries continue to search for broadened support that would lead the Congress to pass a reasonable compromise. And there are a number of additional concerns affecting the rate of federal reimbursement for hospitals and nursing homes on which early action remains problematic.

Moreover, there is little evidence that the broadly supported proposal for early congressional action to limit the number of IMGs admitted to the United States for residency training to no more than 10 percent of the graduates of U.S. medical schools is likely to be debated, much less approved. The support by the American Asso-

ciation of Medical Colleges and the AMA for early and favorable
action by Congress because of their and others' concerns that the
United States may be in, or approaching, a surplus of physicians has
not impressed most members of the Congress. One possible reason
for the continuing relaxed attitude of Congress towards those who
warn of a present or coming physician surplus is the continuing good
record of physician earnings, now approximating $200,000 per an-
num, hardly a precursor of an imminent crisis.

There is broad agreement among the analysts both inside and
outside the Beltway that the health care insurance cycle is definitely
on an upward track with the prospect of revised rates for corporate
health insurance rates returning to double-digit increases. With the
number of uninsured above 40 million and pointing upward; with
managed care plans having withdrawn from a number of markets where they had earlier covered Medicare and/or Medicaid
patients; with excess hospital capacity increasing rather than being eliminated; with no early solution to the introduction of an
effective system of risk adjustment; with the future of many managed care companies uncertain, if not seriously vulnerable, the near-
middle-term outlook for the health care sector must at best be judged
to be uncertain.

One generalization may be safely ventured. The widespread conviction that increasing numbers of employers, investors, and health
administrators developed in the 1980s and early 1990s that for-profit
managed care companies would be able to reform the U.S. health
care sector so as to moderate the long-term rise in the proportion of
the GDP required to maintain a healthy and well-functioning health
care delivery system, at least for all of the insured population, was a
hope and a promise that has not been fulfilled and cannot be fulfilled. The vast majority of Americans continue to look to their physicians for guidance as to the types of care and treatment that they
need and can profit from. Physicians, in turn, undergo the longest
and most arduous period of training of any professional group, and
by law are the only persons authorized to undertake many procedures that can contribute to the patient's future health and well-being, but on occasion can injure or even cause his or her premature
death. It should come as no surprise therefore that patients and physicians, once they recognized the new reality of corporate employers and for-profit managed care companies in close alignment with
each other had stripped more and more health decision-making power

from physicians and patients, would face a rebellion which, in fact, occurred in the latter 1990s.

With the ushering in of the new century, the near-middle- term future of the U.S. health care sector is beset with uncertainties amidst a few realities, such as mounting evidence that managed care companies cannot be relied upon to constrain the future trend of health care expenditures heading toward $2 trillion annual outlay by 2008, or a year earlier or later. At the same time, the last two decades have provided repeated evidence that neither employers nor government can return to the pre-1980 environment when they paid the bills of providers without any, or much, review.

How do the foregoing trends affect the supply of physicians? Since NHE grew by approximately $1 trillion in annual outlays between 1980 and 1999, and since Congress had decided as early as 1976 that the physician shortage had been resolved, the first and most relevant point is that the explosive growth in expenditures did not have more than a marginal influence on the numbers of physicians in the educational pipeline or the numbers that entered practice over the last two decades. But that is not the whole of the story because the five-fold increase in NHE between 1980 and 2000, with a period of modest inflation after 1982, surely contributed to the marked expansion in the number of specialists and subspecialists turned out by the Academic Health Centers and the other teaching hospitals; and the correlated fact that the new entrants were able to establish practices when they had completed their elongated period of residency training; and further were able to command considerably higher incomes than those completing a primary care certification, even considering the stronger demand for the latter as managed care companies employed more of them to serve as gatekeepers.

A second important effect of the much expanded health care financing has to do, as earlier mentioned, with the trend in physicians' incomes. Between 1985 and 1999, the median physician income increased from $94,000 to $170,000 and the average physician's income increased from $112,000 to $200,000. With the sole exception of 1994, when both median and average physician incomes decreased, we have seen a continuous trend of annual increases. As of 1998, the average net income figure showed that hospital-based specialists such as radiologists ($273,400), anesthesiologists ($237,000), and pathologists ($201,000) continue to dominate the ranks of the highest earning physicians, largely as a result of the

Medicare payment system. Primary care physicians, however, have been gaining since they expanded their roles as gatekeepers. In 1996, general and family practitioners were earning on average $139,100. As of 1998, their earnings had increased to $142,000.

An important further clue to the changing dynamic between physician supply and the financing of the health care system relates to the changed incentives facing the members of the medical profession. For the five decades since the end of World War II there was accommodation between the proliferation of specialists and the dominance of the acute care hospital. The hospital offered the specialist a professional environment in which to practice his finely honed skills; and the specialist, in turn, found that he could treat many more seriously ill patients within the hospital where he had ready access not only to the most advanced technology but also to a broad array of support personnel, including residents and fellows, nurses and technicians. The more patients that specialists admitted and treated in a hospital, the larger their earnings and the greater the hospital's revenues.

With the introduction and growth of managed care, however, the incentive structure became radically altered. And despite the uncertain future of managed care companies, the re-connection of dollars and services is not likely to be severed. Physicians who practice in managed care or at least in a cost-conscious environment have a strong incentive to reduce the number of patients that they admit for in-patient care, which is generally far more costly than care provided in other settings. No longer do physicians have an incentive to make heavy use of the hospital. Quite the opposite: in a cost-conscious environment it is to their advantage to contain the numbers whom they hospitalize.

A few additional observations on the interactions between the financing of the health care sector and the trends in the future supply of physicians. We took note earlier of the fact that the large numbers of newly trained specialists and subspecialists found it possible, necessary, and desirable to start practices in suburban areas and in medium-sized communities, which enabled more and more of the public ready access to sophisticated ambulatory and inpatient care close to home, a benefit that they value greatly. However, it had a drawback. During the last quarter of the century, the United States has taken only limited advantage of focusing the care of seriously ill patients in regional centers where the staff has become highly skilled because of the number of patients admitted for specialized care.

A related development reflects the liberal funding for GME: Although the number of graduates from U.S. medical schools has remained substantially unchanged since the early 1980s, at about 16,000 per annum, the fact is that we have allowed a significantly increased number of IMGs to enter U.S. residency programs, the vast majority of whom later on change their temporary visas and enter permanent practice in the United States.

Further, we will delay until chapter 6 the discussion on how the flows of funds into the health care arena affected non-physician clinicians who, in turn, have had some early impacts on the numbers of physicians, impacts that are likely to become more important in the years and decades ahead.

One final observation about health care dollars and the numbers of physicians: The Balanced Budget Act of 1997, which set a target of a $115 billion reduction in prospective payments for Medicare over the five-year time span, 1997-2002, led to increasing criticisms by the leading academic health centers that have warned of the destructive impact of such a reduction on their ability to carry out their multiple missions. Congress took these warnings into account when it moderated the prospective cutbacks in 1999 and 2000. The fact remains, however, that both physicians and dollars are critical for the effective functioning of the nation's health care sector, but even with the much increased number of physicians—a doubling since 1960—and even with a much enlarged flow of funds—four-fold between 1980 and 1999—many individuals, communities, and regions continue to be underserved.

A number of efforts to alter the structure of the institutions that deliver medical care to the American people have been initiated during the last fifteen years, which have in various degrees influenced the mode and style of the way physicians practice. We now turn our attention to these re-organizational efforts.

4

The Acute Care Hospital

The preceding three chapters focused on the central role of physician supply in the provision of health care services to the American people, with special attention focused on the problems of access to and the financing of health care services. In this chapter, we will identify the continuities and changes that have occurred in the structure of health care delivery during the last third of the twentieth century, with a special focus on the central institution, the acute care hospital.

We begin by tracing how the hospital and especially teaching hospitals and the AHCs became the dominant players in health care delivery. For the last fifty years, hospitals have been the centerpiece of medical innovation, medical education, and medical delivery in the United States. More relevant, however, for the purposes of this analysis are the simple facts that who practices medicine, where one practices medicine, with what tools one practices medicine have all depended on the evolution of the acute care hospital. Therefore, essential facets of the changing physician supply question must deal with the challenges that hospitals have faced and will face in the years ahead. How they have responded to these challenges and how these responses might affect future developments and, in turn, help to shape the future of physicians.

Starting in the mid-1960s, the government encouraged hospitals, as we have seen mostly through Medicare funding, to create an environment of medical specialism, never-ending medical innovation, and until recently to enjoy respectable profit margins. That said, we also have witnessed the creation of outpatient clinics, a shift to more outpatient care, challenges of overcapacity, and issues of debt. Managed care entered and put pressure on hospitals for less expensive health care delivery and even though managed care as we have known it may be on its way out, cost pressures continue. Recent attempts at integration either vertical (by buying up home care agencies, physician practices, etc.) or horizontal (networking with other smaller hospitals) were defensive maneuvers on the part of the stronger positioned hospitals to respond to the previously mentioned challenges. Notwithstanding these developments, the acute care hospital does indeed remain the central institution in the American health care delivery sector, albeit changed over the course of the last thirty or so years; and likely to change even more in the years and decades ahead.

1960–1980: A Period of Expansion

After the end of the World War II, the number of community hospitals increased about 30 percent, from 4,444 in 1946 to 5,736 in 1965 and total annual admissions nearly doubled, from 14 million to 27 million. During the next fifteen years, the number of hospitals increased by only a few hundred, the number of hospital beds increased from 741,000 to nearly 1 million, indicating on the one hand the great population growth and on the other the improved access of the elderly and the poor to hospital care under Medicare and Medicaid.

In the fifteen years between 1950 and 1965, the total expenditures of all acute care hospitals increased more than four-fold from $2.1 billion to $9.1 billion annually. By 1980, the figure was just short of $77 billion. After adjusting for inflation, hospital expenditures more than doubled during the second fifteen-year period. The large flows of funds as noted earlier catapulted the acute care hospital and especially the AHCs into a lead position.

Two other trends contributed to this lead position for the nation's hospitals. The first was demographic and the second professional. The 1960s saw a major move towards the suburbs and new smaller metropolitan areas attracting predominantly affluent whites. The new suburbanites, partly because they were accustomed to ready access and partly because their income allowed it, wanted medical care available closer to their new homes. New hospitals began to spring up in the nation's suburbs; and existing hospitals were greatly strengthened. Medical schools in the meanwhile were quick to produce the increased numbers of physicians (in fact, specialists) that these new hospitals needed and wanted. Pathologists, radiologists, surgeons and many other specialists were trained to help staff these new and upgraded suburban hospitals.

During the fifteen years from the passage of Medicare and Medicaid to 1980, bed capacity increased by one-third, from just under 750,000 to approximately 1 million; admissions increased from 19 million to 25.5 million; the occupancy rate and the average length of stay remained more or less constant in the 75 percent range and around eight days, respectively; and the adjusted cost of an in-patient day and a hospital episode increased by 115 percent and 104 percent, respectively. One major development during this period was the sizable expansion in outpatient visits, from 60 million to over 140 million.

1980–2000: Years of Turbulence

During the next twenty years, a number of factors converged to create increasing turmoil in the hospital sector specifically and in the health delivery sector in general. Between 1980 and 1984, the number of admissions remained stable around 25 million annually, but after 1984 the United States experienced a steady decline. Since 1987 admissions never exceeded 22 million despite the growth in both the total population and the cohort of over 75 years old.

Another factor that created problems for the hospital sector was the passage of the prospective payment system (PPS) in 1983 for Medicare. The proponents of the new approach anticipated that it would provide hospitals with a strong incentive to

control their per diem and per episode costs because any savings they realized under the Diagnosis Related Groups (DRGs) schedule were theirs to keep. On the other hand, if they overspent, they would have to absorb the loss. In the first two years of PPS, most hospitals did relatively well; by 1986, however, the initial "overpayment" (an accounting mistake) was eliminated and hospitals faced a much less certain financial future. Oddly enough, large acute care hospitals were able to maintain and even improve their margins once Medicare had replaced cost-based reimbursement with PPS. Instead of moderating their costs of providing care they decided to focus on increasing their total revenues by developing new products. Ambulatory care services, particularly surgery, home health care, women's health services, rehabilitation programs, preventive health programs allowed hospitals to keep increasing their revenue flows. Of course, in doing so each was transforming itself into a larger and different institution than the hospital of the sixties and the seventies.

Some hospitals, however, did not fare well. Two groups of acute care hospitals were most at risk: rural hospitals and voluntary hospitals in the inner cities. Among the reasons that many rural hospitals found themselves in increasing financial turmoil were bed capacity (often below 100 beds), low patient volume due to low population density; inadequate supply of physicians in the community; and the preference of many patients to seek care elsewhere.

The second group of hospitals that faced and, to a degree, still face major financial problems are many urban hospitals located in the inner city, particularly those in areas where the original founders and surrounding communities had moved to the suburbs and been replaced by the inflow of new low-income groups, which suffered from higher morbidity and had fewer resources to pay for medical care. During the 1980s, the inner city of Chicago lost fifteen acute care hospitals. Their increasingly unsatisfactory financial condition reflected declining occupancy, low Medicaid reimbursement, growing numbers of uninsured, tightly managed negotiated rates that lacked the cash flow to sustain such rates, and regionally monitored payments by self-insured employers and commercial firms, which were some of the reasons that inner city hospitals confronted increasing financial turbulence. Oftentimes, hospitals that did not close were sold either to major non-profit institutions or to a for-profit chain, as was the case with Michael Reese Hospital and Medical Center (Chicago), an old teaching hospital that was sold to HUMANA in 1989. Perhaps the most dramatic demise of an inner-city hospital occurred in 1977 in Philadelphia when the city decided to close Philadelphia General Hospital, one of the nation's oldest public hospitals that had served the city's poor for over two centuries.

There were still additional factors that converged during this period to create problems for many hospitals. In recent years, there have been significant underpayments by both Medicare and Medicaid, amounting to roughly 12 percent for the former and 18 percent for the latter. Since the combined payments of Medicare and Medicaid account for 43 percent of all hospital revenues, the underpayments by both programs resulted in a financial emergency for many of the nation's hospitals that were not able to cross-subsidize. By billing private health insurance about 130 percent of the costs actually incurred by their beneficiaries, they were able to cross-subsidize the care provided to Medicare, Medicaid, and uninsured patients. Continuing recourse to cost-shifting, however, was not always possible. In areas of the country with substantial excess hospital capacity and strong managed care delivery systems, the opportunities for substantial cost-shifting had been seriously curtailed, if not eliminated. The strongest managed care companies in Southern California and elsewhere have been able to negotiate discounts as high as 30 to 40 percent from hospitals, in return for an assured number of admissions.

A great many other signs point to major transformations in the hospital sector suggesting that the long established central role of the acute care hospital finds itself under increasing pressure. Since the early 1980s, total inpatient days in hospitals have declined from just under 256 million in 1981 to just under 226 million in 1990, despite an expanding population. In 1998, the number of inpatient days stood at a low of 195 million, a 13.8 percent decline since the beginning of the decade. Moreover, total admissions per 1,000 population also decreased from 125 in 1990 to 119 in 1998, a 4.2 percent decline.

There is every reason to anticipate that the trends of the last decade will continue. In the future, it is reasonable to assume that patients will be admitted for in-patient care only if they are to undergo complex procedures or if they need to be admitted to the intensive care unit. Responding to these trends, community hospitals changed their menu of services. In 1984, less than half of all community hospitals provided outpatient services. By 1993, the rate had risen to just under 94 percent. In 1981, only 3.6 million surgeries were performed in an outpatient setting; in 1991, the figure stood at 11.7 million, an increase of 229 percent within one decade. Furthermore, total outpatient visits increased by 50 percent between 1990 and 1998, from 301 million to 454 million. Clinic visits alone increased at the same time by 68 percent. Also noteworthy was the substantial decline in operations performed in an in-patient setting, from 15.7 million in 1981 to 10.7 million ten years later and to 8.9 million in 1998, a shrinkage of just under 34 percent. This major inversion of the locus of care points to the continuing technological progress in medicine and especially surgery and anesthesiology, as well as to the preference of surgeons to become less dependent on the supporting staff of the in-patient surgical service, and, of course, the reasonable preference of most patients to return home as soon as possible after their encounter with the medical system. And the encouragement of hospital management saw financial benefits from relocating many surgical procedures to the outpatient department, since PPS did not control, at least initially, the rates for Medicare reimbursement for outpatient care. Medicare payments for hospital outpatient care charges increased by 13.4 percent annually between 1984 and 1995, at which time they reached $12 billion.

While the shift in locale for surgical interventions explains much of the growth in the outpatient department, other functions also played a role, such as outpatient rehabilitation. In 1984, these services were provided by only 37 percent of community hospitals; by 1997, the figure stood at over 59 percent. The provision of home health care services also expanded rapidly, from 22 percent to 57 percent of all hospitals. Another growth area of outpatient care was treatment for alcohol and chemical dependency which grew from 14 to 21 percent of all reporting hospitals. Family planning and reproductive health, hospice care, and outpatient services for AIDS patients and for persons requiring psychiatric care provided additional areas of expansion. Many outpatient departments also became involved in providing services for geriatric patients, in some cases even to the home-bound and the institutionalized.

As stated earlier, there are good reasons to assume that the expansion of outpatient services during the past fifteen years will continue in the years ahead. With chronic care becoming one of the most important foci of medical care, as we will see in chapter 5, the need for around-the-clock, ambulatory care will reinforce this trend toward the establishment of outpatient centers in alliance with home health services, including home infusion therapy.

And the recent switch by Medicare to prospective payment for ambulatory care need not deter hospital executives from moving in this direction. Under the new system, Medicare will pay hospitals a fixed amount for each one of about 700 procedural groups. If the hospitals can provide the service and save money, they get to keep it. If they lose money, they have to swallow the loss. Medicare expects to pay this year 4.6 percent more for outpatient care than last year. And since Medicare is the largest single payer, moving more and more services to the outpatient setting is a trend that is likely to keep expanding. The American Hospital Association, on the other hand, estimates a reduction in total outpatient payments of about $9 billion to a level of $74 billion. But overall this does not seem to deter hospital executives. The association budgets a small percentage decline in outpatient payments for the first time since the new system got started and is preparing its member hospitals to be better able to cope with the new system. The potential for better coping exists. Under the old system, emergency room visits were being charged at the minimum code. Not anymore. Many/most hospitals are preparing themselves to take advantage of the pending changes. Despite the shift to prepayment, it seems that the trend towards more ambulatory care will continue.

Other factors, however, especially in the in-patient care arena, present challenges that acute care hospitals will be forced to confront. The first is the continuing steep decline in hospital occupancy rates. Occupancy rates are down since the beginning of the 1990s by almost 5 percent (67 percent in 1990, 62 percent in 1998). That means that local hospitals in a significant number of cities have occupancy rates in the 50 percent range (Los Angeles and Phoenix being the two most prominent examples).

While there are obvious benefits for a community to try to keep its hospitals operating—considering the multiple contributions that hospitals make to the community's economic development, employment, and morale—the costs of gross overcapacity cannot be ignored much longer.

Reference must also be made to the managed care industry, which, despite its own serious problems, has demonstrated the following. Health dollars and services will not be again disconnected and hospital practices will continue to be closely scrutinized. Because of the high costs associated with in-patient care (the average per diem cost was approximately $1,300 in 1998), HMOs and other managed care plans have long sought to avoid unnecessary admissions of their members. As new and different managed care plans expand, efforts to avoid unnecessary hospitalization are certain to grow. Consider California: the stronger managed care plans in Southern California have succeeded in reducing their hospitalization rates for enrollees below 65 years of age to around 180 days per 1,000 as opposed to a national average that is in the 295-day range. Here is one further indicator that the acute care hospital system is likely to be hard-pressed to shrink its much over-expanded capacity.

Hospitals during the last decade or so have adopted the mantra that size matters and through institutional realignments (mergers, networks, and affiliations) have sought to expand in order to increase their referrals and in-patient census. Their micro-management mentality can be summarized as follows: many hospitals want to manage risk fully, develop clinical guidelines, develop regional primary care networks, and improve their system's information system.

Affiliations among hospitals, physician practices, outpatient centers, and other providers have two attractive potentials: first, the ability to subspecialize a number of high-cost treatment modalities with corresponding potential gains in cost control and quality improvements; and second, serving as a strong defense against what hospitals consider to be unreasonable demands from the managed care sector, one of whose principal tactics has been—and if afforded the opportunity will continue to be—to redirect a high volume of their previous hospital admissions to alternative institutions unless hospitals meet their terms for reduced rates.

Only the future will reveal more fully many of the underlying difficulties and dangers that arise from the affiliation—merger movements that are underway. But if the last few years' experience attests to anything it is that the formation of new hospital systems proved not to be the panacea that hospital managers anticipated. Early on most of the key players decided that doing nothing was much riskier than entering into alliances aimed at achieving greater scale and attaining market dominance as the preferred response to the increasingly destabilized marketplace.

In seeking to draw a trial balance sheet after these years of efforts to speed affiliations, networking, and mergers, the following are among the early, if not the permanent, consequences of the organizational realignments that have dominated the recent past. Even in the absence of asset mergers with consequent full integration between the dominant hospital leader and the smaller institutions that joined the larger system, the new affiliations usually provided a small number of cost reducing opportunities to the merged institutions, including joint purchasing of medical supplies and equipment to combining such routine services as laundry, security, accounting, and other critical services.

There is a second area of potential mutual gain to both the larger and the smaller partner following such affiliations. The smaller, often a suburban outlying institution that joins a major AHC system is encouraged to refer selected patients for consultation and treatment to the larger center where the staff is often more experienced and better supported with new technology to provide improved diagnostic and therapeutic interventions. But with most larger suburban hospitals staffed with an array of specialists and even subspecialists, it would be an error to assume that the number of patient referrals from outlying institutions to the dominant center accounts for more than a few percentage points change in the patient census of the receiving hospital per week, per month, or per year. An associated factor that may also create certain benefits especially for the smaller partner is related to the willingness of the center to assign residents and supervisory staff to the smaller institution.

But having identified these potential benefits to both partners arising out of networking and mergers, one must stop to note the limits to fuller integration that might be achieved by closing services such as duplicating specialties or taking even more radical action such as closing the smaller, outlying institution in a market area that may be suffering from substantial excess capacity. Aside from the communal responsibility of the trustees to assure that their institution continues to provide essential services to the local population, there are several other important forces that will usually fight hard against institutional extinction—the professional staff whose livelihood is linked to the continued use of the hospital and the sizable numbers of hospital employees who stand to lose their jobs and income if their institution ceases to operate. And to complicate matters even more, many small hospitals may be carrying a heavy mortgage debt, leaving the board of trustees in a vulnerable position in the case of default.

If our contention is valid, that the hospital sector is characterized by substantial excess in-patient capacity; and continuing shifts are still underway from acute to chronic care; and from in-patient to ambulatory treatment settings then it follows that the challenges to networks and affiliations fall short of the shrinkage and elimination of in-patient capacity that the future market demand still requires.

This conclusion emerges from the recent Delloitte and Touche hospital survey entitled *2000 U.S. Hospitals and the Future of Health Care Survey*. A growing number of hospital CEOs expect their hospitals to remain free-standing, while only a few years earlier, in 1994, less than one in five CEOs made such a forecast. In fact, this survey supports the argument that a majority of CEOs would rather restructure and eliminate clinical services, downsize facilities and lay-off staff instead of pursuing a merger.

The last two decades have provided a sizable number of innovations and experiments aimed at altering the ways in which the health care sector is organized; and how the two principal providers of medical care—hospitals and physicians—produce and deliver the care that patients seek and are able and willing to pay for. Even today, 80 percent of physician groups in the United States have only between three and nine physicians. This modest scale of practice arrangements underscores the constrained opportunities that exist for any short-term radical reorganization as to how physicians deliver medical care.

Admittedly, this largely cottage-based arrangement could be altered and on occasion has been altered but with equivocal results. The last two decades have seen aggressive efforts made by leading hospitals and academic health centers to purchase physician practices in the hope and expectation that a much-expanded medical enterprise consisting of a major teaching hospital, a much-expanded physician staff of both primary care physicians and specialists and subspecialists all belonging to the same health care enterprise, under a single management structure, would lead to more effective and more efficient outcomes for the patients who sought treatment and better outcomes, as well for the system and its providers.

An attractive theory, but it is difficult to find many examples of such expansionary efforts having proved themselves. A major drawback relates to the maintenance of physicians' practice efforts, once the ownership of the practice has been transferred from the individual physician or small group to the new and expanded centralized system.

A greater dependence on "competition," likewise developed a reputation for efficiency and effectiveness which later experience failed in part or whole to support. In the absence of any effective risk adjustment mechanism to take into account the needs of potentially high-cost patients, most physician groups have been reluctant to enter into capitation agreements with managed care plans.

A decade or so ago when the managed care revolution was still accelerating it appeared that a likely change might occur through the formation of PHOs (physician-hospital organizations) that would conjointly design an integrative approach to attract and treat patients, both ambulatory and in-patients, within a single organizational framework. Although one can point to such selected efforts succeeding, the more striking fact is that they have been relatively few and far between. It is easier to foresee the potential gains that might be achieved from such cooperative undertakings than to fashion a new organization that can develop the track record that produces gains.

Another potential for change that has remained more potential than reality: Within almost every health care market characterized by substantial excess hospital capacity one would have expected considerable entrepreneurial efforts aimed at mergers, buyouts, closures leading to a removal of excess beds. While some hospitals were bought, merged, or closed, the striking fact is that in most larger communities there has been very little and often no closure of any sizable hospital, among other reasons because of the importance of the institution to the local inhabitants for medical care, for jobs, for income; and the further fact that if the institution carries substantial debt, as so many do, it will not be attractive to potential buyers. And not to be overlooked are the efforts that the physician staff, or at least most members, are likely to exert on trustees to keep the hospital open. One must not overlook the fact that the predominant number of teaching and community hospitals operate under nonprofit or governmental auspices, which means that the responsible leadership will explore almost any and all alternatives before agreeing to close their institution.

Into the New Century—What Lies Ahead?

As one looks ahead to the first decades of the new century, a showdown may result from the unsettling developments of important provider systems on both the East and West Coasts and places in between, developments that reflect failed efforts to constrain costs and often led to future cost increases. Just consider the troubles facing Beth Israel Hospital in Boston, as well as the earlier bankruptcy of the area's Pilgrim Health Insurance Plan. In New York City, the most attractive of the for-profit managed care companies, Oxford, all but collapsed early in 1997 and is not yet fully recovered. Aetna, the largest of the for-profit insurance companies recently dismissed its chief executive and its stock is considerably off from its highest level. In Philadelphia, there have been two warning developments—the bankruptcy of the Allegheny Health Care System and the subsequent indictment of several of its senior executives; and the horrendous financial setback of the Pennsylvania University Health Care System in 1999, which reported losses of about $200 million for the year, attesting to the fact that management's ambitious plans to erect a well-functioning delivery system including both a large group of primary care physicians up to the highest levels of subspecialty care, with an optimal patient treatment plan was easier to sketch out than to turn into a reality.

On the West Coast, one can point to the unhappy outcome of the efforts of the two leading academic health centers, Stanford and the University of California, San Francisco, to coordinate selected clinical activities to avoid unnecessary duplication and wasteful expenditures, a well-intended effort that floundered in execution. There is no need to look elsewhere to identify additional efforts at reform that failed to meet the expectations of the reformers. The hospital sector seems to be struggling along with its accumulated troubles and only two trends appear to be confirmed: in-patient services are increasingly being shifted to an out-patient basis; and prospective payments or capitation seem to be the predominant mode of paying for hospital care.

How have physicians been affected by these changes? Consider the following: First, in terms of practice, physicians have lost part of their autonomy and are striving to get it back. To the extent, however, that dollars and services will from now on remain connected, a reasonable assumption, physicians will not regain all of their former autonomy. The question is, who will share it? Possibly physician associations or AHCs or hospital and physician groups will jointly assume more risk and more responsibility to sustain the medical delivery system. If one or another of these developments occurs, physicians may be able to regain a large part of their lost control over the medical delivery system. But this would challenge physicians to put in place and manage health care resources more prudently. Second, physicians today find themselves practicing in increasingly diverse settings (hospitals, clinics, private practices, etc.) because of managerial changes that hospitals in general and AHCs specifically have made. Also they confront a growing number of other professionals who also have clinical skills, albeit not as many as physicians (nurse practitioners, nurses, physician assistants). At the same time, the population at risk as we will explore in the next chapter, will need a broadened menu of types of care (acute, chronic, home, etc.), which doctors and NPCs working jointly will need to provide. Physician supply policy and health management will have to take these trends and approaches into consideration in altering the delivery of medical care as a continuum in which an enlarged number of professionals interact with the patient and with one another.

Finally, the question arises what kind of physicians should medical schools prepare? How best can tomorrow's physicians be provided with the clinical skills they will need? In what settings? Will the AHCs be able to respond to these challenges? Or will institutional inertia and specialty conflicts slow or prevent their adjustment to the changing U.S. health care marketplace? These are questions that a dynamic policy must address and resolve. The challenges that loom ahead are increasingly clear. The alternative solutions must still be developed.

5

Aging and the Future of U.S. Health Care

Even a casual observer of the changing United States cannot help but be impressed by the strong effects that demographic trends and changes over the years have had on the nation's health care system in general and on the medical personnel supply changes which responded at least in part to these trends. The doubling of physician supply that got underway in 1963, which was aimed primarily at accommodating the increased demand, especially in the suburbs where many people had relocated, is a potent reminder of this fact. Demography is once again destined to present the overall health care system and society in general with major challenges, as we move forward towards 2030. With the first four chapters of the volume focused on how physician supply interacted with the acute care system, this chapter will focus on one of the major challenges that American society will face, the doubling of its elderly population between 2010 and 2030, from 35 million to over 70 million.

Aging, especially among the post-85 age group, carries with it many unpleasant concomitants, such as a reduced capacity of many individuals to deal effectively with the demands of independent living, which include not only the continuing physical and mental capacity to control one's life but also to do so in a fashion that enables the individual to derive pleasure and satisfaction from the ways in which he or she is able to continue meaningful relations with relatives and friends. No person, young, middle aged, or old, can live a meaningful life cut off from other persons.

The aging of the baby boom generation presents the United States with two distinct challenges. The first relates to the expansion of medical care (acute care and chronic care) required to meet the needs of much larger numbers. The second is focused on "maintenance support." Maintenance support is not medical care and should not be confused with it, although many of the elderly require both. We will consider maintenance support in the chapter that follows.

All demographic models point up that the United States will face an aging crisis. According to conservative estimates, the number of people over 65 will double by 2030. Having recognized that aging often leads to a reduction in physical, mental, and social attributes required to enable the older person (as well as some seriously handi-capped younger persons) to function effectively without the help of others—family, friends, neighbors, and hired help—the critical ques-tion that this chapter addresses deals with the changes confronting our society as the numbers of the elderly, and especially the above-85 contingent, will double and quadruple over the next decades and the corresponding adjustments that such an aging trend will require in the practices of the medical profession and the health care sector.

We begin, by exploring the current sites for providing care to the elderly, pointing out that there are three settings where such care is provided. Most acute or chronic medical care is provided in ambu-latory care settings under the control of hospitals or physicians, and in acute care hospitals. Much of the care that patients receive in nursing homes or at home has less to do with medical care rendered by physicians or non-physician clinicians but consists of support services that the patients require to cope with the demands that they face in daily living. Increasingly, a number of patients who require support to cope with their requirements for daily living have opted to live at home.

Looking back since the implementation of Medicare and Medic-aid, a third of a century ago, it should be clear that very substantial new funding was made available by the federal government to broaden and deepen access for the sick elderly for acute care treat-ment, largely hospital based. Secondarily, Medicaid funding was heavily focused on the elderly suffering from chronic illness, in-cluding those who require a shorter or longer admission to a nursing home. And during the past decade both Medicaid and Medicare have devoted more funding to help care for the many sick and infirm living at home.

By way of helping the reader to recognize some of the challenges that the United States will face as it confronts a sizable increase—more than a doubling of persons over 65 years of age in the decades ahead, and an even greater rate of increase in the old elderly, those

85 or above—we need to focus on the fact that while many/most of the elderly will require continuing access to acute care services, they will also require much more attention in helping them cope with chronic illness.

The relative growth and increased prevalence of chronic illness among the older population helps to highlight among other questions whether there may be more reliance in the future on the roles of non-physician clinicians, particularly nurse practitioners, nurses and physician assistants, who might assume a large part of the burden of making home visits to the chronically ill who have limited or no mobility.

No matter how skeptical one may be about forecasts made at the beginning of the twenty-first century about events a quarter of a century or further into the future, there is no reason to challenge the assumptions that the United States will face by 2030 at least a doubling of the number of persons 65 and older, and a significantly larger number of persons over 85. Further, there is no reason to challenge the forecast that an older population will need more medical attention and treatment, even if physicians will, in many if not in most encounters, be unable to restore the patient to full functioning.

Current Data of the Care of the Elderly

A close look at the average annual expenditure for health care per consumer unit provides some important insights. Consider the following:

- The two lowest quartiles spend between 7.3 and 7.7 percent of their income for health care while those in the top twentieth income class spend just under 4 percent (3.9). As the number of the elderly increase, we can expect an increased financial burden on those lower on the income scale.

- During the period 1980 to 1996, a significant increase occurred in the number of physician contacts by patients belonging to different age groups. There was practically no change in the number of visits except between the two highest age groups, those between 45 and 64 from 5.1 to 7.2 visits, and the more striking change in the 65 and above group that had an increase of contacts from 6.4 to 11.7 over the same time period.

- In 1997, the number of visits to office-based physicians was 3, and the age group 45 to 64 had only a slightly higher number—3.5 visits. But the two subgroups 65 to 74 and 75 and over averaged, respectively, 5.5 and 6.5 visits.

But the data just reviewed about the increases in patient visits to physicians is only the beginning, not the end in an assessment as to the likely impacts that the aging of the U.S. population will have on the nation's health care system in the decades ahead.

Acute Care

The above-65 population, roughly 13 percent of the U.S. population, accounts at the beginning of the twenty-first century for about forty percent of all acute care hospital expenditures ($179 billion), which represented about 13 percent of NHE. The predominant sources of payment for acute care hospital costs for the elderly are in the first instance Medicare and secondarily Medicaid, with all other sources of payment accounting for a very small percentage of the total.

Further, special note needs to be taken of the fact that elderly persons make much greater use of in-patient hospital facilities than do those in the younger age brackets. Among those 45 to 64 years of age 117 of each 1,000 patients discharged fell into this age bracket. But among those 65 to 74 the proportion was more than double, 257 per 1,000; and among those 75 years and over the proportion rose to 455 per 1,000 or about four times greater than the 45 to 64 age group. What these data underscore is the heavy use that the elderly population makes of high-tech medicine and the most sophisticated medical care interventions.

It is equally striking that in terms of the principal areas of treatment there are only minor differences among the several age groups in terms of first-listed diagnoses which in every middle and older age group are focused on diseases of the heart, malignant neoplasm, injuries and poisoning, cerebrovascular disease, and in the two oldest age groups, pneumonia.

While there have been, as noted below, some modest adaptations of the U.S. health care system during the last several decades to the growing numbers of the elderly, the leaders of the medical establishment as well as its principal institutions—medical schools, academic health centers, and the biomedical research sector—have continued down the path on which they started out shortly after World War II to push back the frontiers of high-tech medical treatment for the sick and injured with primary focus on acute care treatment for all patients admitted to teaching and community hospitals.

The best evidence of this continuing focus of U.S. medicine on acute care treatments for all insured persons, including the elderly, was the passage of Medicare in 1965 which assured that the above-65 population would continue to have access to mainline physician and hospital care even if they were no longer covered by private health insurance providers as they had been prior to their retirement. Medicare, when it was implemented in 1966, however, paid little if any attention to the large numbers of the elderly who needed diagnostic and therapeutic assistance to help them manage one or more chronic conditions. Neither the leaders of the medical profession nor the principal teaching hospitals evinced much interest in assessing the needs of the growing numbers of patients with chronic conditions, much less in treating them.

But one must be careful not to overstate the case because in the succeeding decades a limited number of medical centers sought to respond to the growing numbers of patients with chronic conditions that called for redefinitions and adjustments in their prior almost exclusive focus on high-tech medicine directed to curing patients with acute conditions.

Since we have dealt extensively in the earlier chapters with the ongoing preoccupation of U.S. medicine with high-tech advances and the improved delivery of acute care services, we will focus the remainder of this chapter on medical and related support services provided the elderly other than in acute care hospitals—specifically in nursing homes and via home care programs.

Nursing Homes

As to nursing homes, the current census totals approximately 1.5 million residents over the age of 65, with half being released within a six months' span, but with 7 percent remaining on the rolls, some for as long as five years. Just about half of all patients received help with bathing and dressing, with a substantial proportion of patients also requiring assistance in transferring from bed to chair, preparing meals, using the toilet and similar tasks. The dominant services provided, in descending order, are nursing services (84 percent), physical therapy (20 percent), social services and medications, each about 10 percent. Household services were provided to 28 percent of all patients, but physician services and nutrition services were provided to less than 4 percent. About nine out of every ten residents have to use a wheelchair or a walker; and one out of every four has a vision or hearing impairment. What is more, between two-thirds and three-quarters need assistance in the essential activities of daily living such as taking care of their personal possessions and managing their money.

As early as 1973, Congress amended the Medicaid statute to make it possible for the poor and the near poor to be admitted to nursing homes for routine care, with the government (federal and state) paying the bills. It should be emphasized that this new Medicaid funding policy encouraged many for-profit enterprises to enter the nursing home arena and to expand the existing capacity by orders of magnitude, aimed at caring not only for patients who were Medicaid eligible but also to provide expanded nursing home capacity to care for additional patients able to pay out-of-pocket.

Because of the small number of the population that carries insurance for nursing home care, however, the two most prevalent sources of payment are Medicaid for patients who earlier spent down to very low limits of wealth and income to qualify for government funding, and out-of-pocket payments by the family. In descending order, Medicaid is responsible for 44 percent of total outlays; family support or out-of-pocket payments account for another 31 percent. Medicare provides 14 percent and private insurance 7 percent with the small residual coming from other sources. Specialists in Social Security and pensions have repeatedly called attention to the need for reform especially as regards additional retirement payments being available to surviving widows (see *Social Security: Out of Step with the Modern Family*, Urban Institute, 2000).

In the mid-1990s, there were just under 1.7 million elderly persons resident in nursing homes, with a striking difference between the sexes with females accounting for three out of every four residents, a reflection of two facts: females, on average, have a life span several years longer than males, and most married women survive their husbands. The predominant proportion of nursing home residents are between 75 and 84, or 85 years and older, these two high age groups accounting for more than eight out of ten nursing home residents. The predominant number (close to 80 percent of nursing home residents) were admitted either from a hospital or from their private residence; the remainder were transfers from another nursing home, a board and care facility, or a retirement home.

The last decade has seen, however, a modest decline in the number of patients being cared for in nursing homes, a consequence of several trends. The typical cost of a yearly stay is currently around $40,000 and in the better staffed and operated institutions the annual cost is often considerably higher, circa $60,000 or even more. Further, it has proved quite difficult for the states to establish and enforce a set of quality requirements that all nursing homes must meet. But the key factor in recent trends in moderating the nursing home census has been the marked preference of most chronically ill patients not to be separated from their families and neighbors and forced to relocate and adjust to a new setting, with new rules, and become dependent on new caregivers.

Home Care

An interesting observation about the above-65 population is their differential use of in-patient hospital services versus home health care services during the 1990-97 years. During this period, there was a substantial decline in covered days of hospital care per admission from 8.9 days at the beginning of the decade to 6.5 in 1997, a decline of about 30 percent. During the same period, the number of enrollees served by home health services approximately doubled. The point is not that home care or chronic care will replace acute care but rather that both types of care will be very much needed in the future.

Furthermore, it is critically important to note that family members and friends account for the predominance of the care provided to patients cared for at home. Further, with women and adult children traditionally carrying most of the responsibility for providing such care, with a high proportion of elderly women living alone, having survived their husbands, and with an increasing proportion of children living in cities other than those of their parents or parent, the challenge of care-giving becomes that much more difficult, more so since about 1:3 of all care-givers, mostly women, are themselves elderly. One response to this challenge of geographic separation between adult children and a surviving parent has been for some of the latter to relocate sooner or later to the home of one of their children, an alternative that is not, however, always available or welcomed.

Recognizing, therefore, the preference of most patients to remain at home, or at least in their community where they have long resided, and the challenges that care-givers confront, a growing number of states have made it possible for many low-income elderly to be cared for at home with Medicaid picking up all or part of the costs.

Further, Medicare recognized in the 1980s that it might speed the early release of certain patients from acute care hospitals if it provided some home-based specialized care services to speed their recovery. But, in 1989, Medicare went further and established a broad-based home care benefit for its enrollees that included not only medical services but also assistance for personal care. As a consequence of such broadened coverage, the home health care benefit outlays for Medicare increased from $3.6 billion in 1990 to over $20 billion by 1997. Between 1990 and 1997, the number of Medicare enrollees participating in Home Health Care more than doubled, from 1.8 million to almost 3.7 million. As a consequence of the Balanced Budget Act of 1997, Medicare initiated a series of reforms to moderate the earlier steep rise in its home care benefit costs to a point where its expenditure level declined by the end of 1999 to $19 billion, with possible modifications in the program aimed at further reductions. Even more striking than the above cited doubling in the number of patients enrolled in Medicare Home Health Care coverage was the more than five-fold increase in per capita expenditure during the decade, which underlies the reasons for the BBA cuts for home care. It should be noted that these recent changes in federal financing policies have resulted in considerable upheaval in the home care industry, most of which operates in the for-profit sector with many companies finding it impossible to absorb the recent cutbacks in federal financing and forced to cease operations.

A sub-summary follows of the presentation up to this point, which has focused on the implications of the prospective aging of the U.S. population, more particularly the prospective doubling of the above-65 year olds between 2011 and 2030. If past is prologue, the aging of the U.S. population will result in a doubling of the above-65 population in the two decades between 2011 and 2030, with many living into their eighties and nineties and even longer. However, the growing number of the elderly will require both acute and chronic care and a minority will be so severely handicapped that they will be cared for in nursing homes. A great many others will prefer to continue to live at home or in assisted living arrangements in their community where a significant proportion suffering from advanced chronic conditions will require considerable assistance in helping them cope with the challenges of daily living.

What follows are the more important findings that we were able to extract from our review of recent trends in the U.S. health care sector that must be included in any effort to assess what the near future may hold in store.

Andrew Cohen, in an article in *Academic Medicine*, noted, "The growing predominance of chronic illness will be the major challenge facing the American health care system in the coming century. Patients with chronic conditions account for three-fourths of U.S. health care expenditures." This point is supported by the following trend data. Whereas in 1900 deaths in the United States from cardiovascular disease and cancer accounted for 20.1 and 3.7 percent, in 1990, the respective rates were 42 percent and 23.2 percent. Technologies such as coronary angioplasty, thrombolytic therapy, and chemotherapy have allowed patients to survive ischemic heart disease and neoplasia and converted these diseases from acute to chronic conditions. In 1996, chronic illness accounted for more than three-fourths of all U.S. health care expenditures ($659 billion). Furthermore, patients who have a chronic condition account for 80 percent of hospital days, 69 percent of hospital admissions, 66 percent of physician visits, and 55 percent of emergency room visits. In terms of chronic care, they require 96 percent of home care visits and 83 percent of prescription drug care.

It is also true that most hospitalized patients admitted and treated for heart disease or cancer together account for roughly two-thirds of all admissions to acute care hospitals. When discharged at the end of their treatment they are more likely than not to confront one or more chronic conditions for which there are no known cures but only ameliorative interventions. Reworded, this means that with an ever-growing number of the population living into their seventies and eighties and even longer, the medical care that more and more patients will require in the second and third decades of the twenty-first century must provide access to both acute and chronic care.

But even in the face of a growing shift from in-patient to ambulatory care sites, the acute care hospital with its army of specialists, sophisticated technology, and extended support staff, from nurses to technicians, continues to provide the major center of American medicine's interventions and therapeutic accomplishments. The present preoccupation of U.S. medicine, as emphasized earlier, remains overwhelmingly to seek new and better means of treating and curing patients who present acute care conditions. That is how most medical students are instructed by their professors in medical school and, further, how most residents are prepared during their residency training before becoming licensed to practice medicine. As noted earlier, about 31.6 million patients were treated in the nation's community hospitals in 1997; and their average length of stay came to 6.1 days, down from 7.6 days in 1980, which marked the turning point in the long-term upward trend in admissions for in-patient care. In 1997, hospital expenditures both in-patient and ambulatory continued to account for the single largest sub-sector of the nation's health care expenditures, which in that year totaled just under $1.1 trillion. Although there has been a pronounced decline in the share of hospital expenditures after 1980 as a percentage of national health expenditures (NHE), from 42 to 34 percent of the total, hospital care still dominates the rapidly increasing NHE which exceeded $1 trillion in 1997, up from slightly under $250 billion in 1980. Even with this relative steep decline in the proportion of acute care hospital outlays by the latter 1990s, it is important to note that hospital expenditures were about three times greater than the institutional outlays for the care of chronic patients with nursing home outlays totaling $83 billion and home health care outlays reaching $32 billion.

Furthermore, a little appreciated but important fact alluded to above but which now warrants emphasis is the peripheral role that physicians play in the direct care of patients in nursing homes, less than 4 percent of whom receive treatment from physicians. And physicians are also often conspicuous by their absence from attending patients receiving home health care services. "The predominant care-givers for chronically ill patients are not physicians but rather nurses, nurses' aides, mental health workers, case managers, social workers, nonprofessionals including family and friends," writes Cohen. Nevertheless, physicians play the key role in managing the illnesses, developing strategies for control of symptoms, following the progression of the illnesses, and dealing with the end stages of dying and death.

A more cautious formulation of Cohen's observations would be that physicians should assume the above responsibilities, but currently seldom do so. In 1998, physicians accounted for 740,000 of the approximately 4 million health care professionals involved in diagnosis and treatment, amounting to 1:5 of all health professionals, or slightly under 6.5 percent of total employment in the health care sector. But they do not constitute the fastest growing profession. In 1996, the U.S. Department of Labor developed a ten-year projection (1996-2006) of the largest and the fastest growing health occupations, which included the following. Three groups of medical employees were estimated to be among the fastest growing occupations: home health aides and nursing aides, orderlies and attendants, and medical assistants:

Personal and Home Care Aides
Physical and Curative Therapy Assistants
Home Health Aides
Medical Assistants
Physical Therapists
Occupational Therapist Assistants

Occupational Therapists
Medical Research Technicians
Spanish Language Pathologists
Dental Hygienist
Physicians Assistants
Emergency Medical Technicians
Dental Assistants

What is most striking about the foregoing listing is that the health care sector accounts for fifteen out of the thirty fastest growing occupations in the projected time period of 1996-2006.

The challenges that the U.S. health care system, as well as the systems of other advanced nations face in the twenty-first century as a consequence of the aging of their populations, will not be easy to confront and resolve. The remainder of this chapter will point to potential responses to the challenges that will confront the United States, health care delivery system in the period after 2011 when the first of the baby boom generation will reach retirement age; and further when the numbers and proportion of the more elderly population, above 75 and above 85 years of age, are expected to undergo large absolute and relative increases in their numbers. Relatively conservative estimates point to the above-85 population growing from around 1 percent of the population at present to 4 percent by 2030.

What follows is a discussion of an alternative model of caring for the elderly. It is called the model On-Lok program and has been replicated by the nine PACE (Program of All-Inclusive Care for the Elderly) sites. On-Lok is based on a continuum of care and capitated payments. Its premise is to have nursing home eligible clients receive integrated services through adult day health centers. Case management and integrated funding are the key, thereby helping to keep the elderly in the community. Proving cost effective care is essential to expanding the financing of these programs. The program (provider) assumes financial risk by accepting capitated Medicare and Medicaid reimbursement. However, many potential clients view the closed network as a drawback and will not join because they do not want to lose their freedom to choose their own providers. The use of multidisciplinary teams to evaluate potential clients for acceptance into a program and determining care plans are another important aspect of the program, as is attendance at the adult day health centers where much of the primary medical care is delivered. Transportation to and from the centers is provided. For programs to remain financially viable, keeping hospital utilization under control becomes crucial. Home health services are available to clients when deemed necessary by the multidisciplinary team, as are homemaker and personal care services; rehabilitative services are provided at the health centers.

Family support is viewed as critical to the success of the On-Lok (and PACE) model. There is a broad reliance on family members as caregivers. When this is not possible, certain sites provide a housing option. Some clients and providers consider this latter effort controversial since it challenges the central idea of "keeping the elderly in their community setting." Redefining the concept of home is one of the foundations of expanding community Long Term Care (LTC). Groups stressing this delivery mode believe that private residences are not the only venue appropriate for home-based care. It can include group living situations such as adult foster homes and group residential settings. In these facilities housekeeping functions and personal care responsibilities remain separate. "Assisted living" complexes (apartments) offer another alternative. Both client and families welcome the availability of an unfurnished self-contained unit with bathroom and kitchen and keys to lock their unit. This, in conjunction with a facility that offers a full range of personal care, housekeeping and nursing services and a communal dining room, allows people to retain some measure of control over their lives. The key distinction between home care and institutionalized care is the scope for self- determination. In a nursing home setting, residents must live according to the regimen established by the management of the nursing home. At home a person usually exercises his or her legal rights to decide on their treatment plan, pursue other choices and have some say over their caregivers. The foregoing underscores some of the difficulties in drawing rigid distinctions between patients suffering from a chronic disease and patients who might be classified as acute care patients. The foregoing helps to explain why one of the tenets of primary care—continuity of patient care—is as relevant today as ever, if not more so. And that is one of the main reasons that working towards the integration of acute and long-term care is essential.

At the beginning of the twenty-first century in the United States, three major issues in terms of elderly care can be identified without any prescription that effective solutions are at hand or will soon become available.

1. It is highly problematic that the leading academic medical centers and the nation's leading biomedical researchers will in the near/middle term turn away from their long-term focus on high-tech medicine. Moreover, even if one were able to encourage them to shift their focus away from the frontiers of medical knowledge and acute medical interventions in favor of paying more attention to the elderly suffering from chronic diseases it would be a questionable tactic. There is a great deal that we still need to know about how to treat more effectively the acutely sick and injured, and the research laboratory and high-tech hospitals will continue to require long-term support and liberal financing if these prospective goals are to be pursued and achieved.

    But having stipulated that it would be foolish and wrong to turn away from investing additional resources in the discovery and application of new biomedical knowledge for the cure of acute illnesses, it would also be an error not to accelerate, by an order of magnitude, efforts to respond more effectively to the long-term trends in chronic diseases affecting primarily the elderly that have only recently become visible and which have as yet attracted relatively little response.

2. With physicians accounting for fewer than one out of five health care professionals and one out of sixteen persons working in the health care sector, much more attention must be directed to exploring possible changes in the relations of physicians to other health professionals and medical support staff that could contribute to more effective

interventions on behalf of patients suffering from both acute and chronic conditions.

A first challenge relates to possible changes in the medical school curriculum along the following dimensions: selected joint clinical training between medical students and students preparing for nursing; much greater emphasis on expanded training for physicians in ambulatory care settings; and much more exposure of medical and other health care students in training focused on elderly patients living at home and/or in nursing homes. Some programs already operational in Boston University, Stanford, the University of North Carolina, and Washington University are aimed at broadening the experience of medical students and residents to patients with chronic conditions including home visits. Integrating acute and chronic care in medical education would allow students to understand better many diseases' natural history, contribute to closer relationships between clinicians and their patients, and assist in achieving improved care outcomes.

3.   Organizational innovations focused on hospitals and their physician staffs taking the lead and working more closely with nurse and other non-physician clinicians and other health providers should aim to design and implement more effective interventions for non-hospitalized patients with chronic disease, especially those living at home.

The next chapter will focus attention on older persons with chronic conditions, most of whom will continue to live at home, with particular attention to the broadened opportunities that should be expanded for physicians and non-physician clinicians to cooperate more effectively in caring for this rapidly growing population.

6

Physicians and Non-Physician Clinicians: Working Together and Independently

Having established that the United States, will soon face a number of challenges in terms of the aging of its population, both in total numbers as well as the proportion of the elderly over 75, we noted that one of the ways for the improved integration of acute and chronic care to be achieved is through better coordination and cooperation between physicians and other providers of clinical services, especially in the primary care arena. The evolution of the professional categories that together constitute the group known as non-physician clinicians (NPCs), as well as their relationship to the medical profession reflect one of the most interesting innovations in the American supply of medical personnel in recent decades. They also constitute the main focus of this chapter.

We begin by exploring how these "new" professions became part of health care delivery and how they relate to the traditional providers of clinical care, physicians. We then focus on recent trends in their education and their roles as autonomous providers of medical care in their own right, reviewing the debate about the ability of NPCs to be independent providers of care. Finally, we look briefly at how the states are dealing with this issue and seek to identify what the future might hold. Throughout, we build the argument that whereas physicians have to remain the health care professionals with the greatest responsibility for clinical innovations and interventions, NPCs are well situated to care independently for a wide range of patients and provide the linkages among different therapeutic settings so that improved continuity of care can be achieved. Furthermore, a more coordinated approach to medical personnel policy is in order so that we do not reach a point where a surplus of both physicians and NPCs occurs and at the same time important issues of access and financing have not been effectively tackled and resolved.

At this point, we need to define once again non-physician clinicians. They include practitioners trained in chiropractic medicine, naturopathy, and acupuncture. Such disciplines are generally regarded as unconventional or alternative to the practice of allopathic or osteopathic medicine practiced by a physician. However, there are other non-physician clinicians whose disciplines are more closely related to the mainline practice of medicine. Three such examples are the nurse practitioner, the physician assistant, and the certified nurse midwife. More specifically, there are ten professional groups that are included in the term non-physician clinician. These are nurse practitioners, certified nurse midwives, physician assistants, chiropractors, acupuncturists, naturopaths, optometrists, podiatrists, certified registered nurse anesthetics, and clinical nurse specialists. We will focus this chapter on how the three subgroups that are most closely involved in medical practice can work more effectively with physicians to improve the quality of care available to the American people. These three professions are nurse practitioners (NP), certified nurse-midwives (CNM), and physician assistants (PA), which together are known as the traditional NPCs.

NPCs emerged at a time when there was a perceived shortage of physicians in the United States, particularly in rural areas. Thus, they were originally employed to serve as physician substitutes, but over the years, they have evolved practice modes that offer patients a distinctive approach to health care. The first NPCs came from the nursing profession, but today the three key groups tend to be graduates of educational programs that have differentiated themselves from nursing. The nurse practitioner (NP), the physician assistant (PA), and the certified nurse midwife (CNM) are nursing-related specialists. Practitioners of all three disciplines must complete clinical training and sometimes post-graduate study to be licensed to practice. The NP and the PA are trained to provide primary care. The key distinction between the two is that the PA is trained to work under the supervision of a physician, while the NP is not. Still, they generally offer the same range of services. The CNM is the modern day practitioner of midwifery, a discipline that has existed since antiquity. Today, midwifery has been incorporated as a specialty of nursing, but there are still a few lay-midwives in active practice. Due to the overlapping of these three disciplines with medicine, physicians have generally been opposed to the independence of these new physician clinicians. Granting them independence could be a threat to physicians' livelihoods, the more so since an NP, PA, or CNM usually charges a lower fee than a physician.

In the past, strong physician lobbies have been able to limit the ability of many NPCs to practice independently. Physicians have successfully influenced policymakers to act in their favor, but physicians today do not enjoy the same status and political influence that they enjoyed in the 1970s. Although they continue to have a central role in the shaping of U.S. health care, they no longer dominate the much-expanded health care delivery system. The growing concern of the American public about health care costs and the public's growing openness to explore alternative methods of health care delivery must be considered. NPCs may soon gain the ability to practice independently of physicians. At no point, however, should the two disciplines sever all ties since the coordination of their services is essential for the improved integration of acute and chronic care as well as for greater continuity of care.

In raising demands for greater independence, NPCs have found themselves, in turn, in intensified battles with physicians. It is worth recalling that the initial impetus for the development of NPCs came originally from the medical profession, many of whose leaders may not have fully appreciated that their actions (expanding the training of physician assistants) might lead to a new professional group that could challenge the physician's central role in medical care delivery.

The Push for More Physician Assistants and Its Unintended Consequences

One of the most interesting events in the history of U.S. health care has been the rise in the economic power and social status of the American physician in the twentieth century. For much of this past century, American physicians have held a place in society above that of their predecessors as well as their colleagues in other parts of the world. In the post-World War II decades, they were able to become the dominant and controlling force in shaping the future of U.S. health care. In the latter half of the twentieth century, physicians not only dominated the U.S. health care system, but also achieved economic power. As a result, the practice of health care by non-physician clinicians was viewed as threatening by many physicians and was met with formidable opposition. Unless the medical profession had decided that it needed to expand the supply of NPCs, a supply that it would, of course, control, the rapid growth of the new practices would have been unlikely.

Before the twentieth century, there was a lack of effective medical treatments that physicians could implement. In addition, there was no standard design for medical school training, and the practice of medicine was largely unscientific. These conditions started to change early on in the twentieth century. Scientific methods were introduced into medicine, and medical education became increasingly standardized. In addition, effective treatments for selected illnesses were developed. These changes became increasingly prominent by the time of World War II. By then, most Americans accepted physicians as the authority on health care. Physicians had increasingly strong claims to authority. They were knowledgeable about the course of many illnesses and they had intimate contact with sick or injured individuals often on a daily basis. The fact that many patients were often seriously ill and in pain provided additional acceptance and support of the physician's judgment. As new technology and pharmaceuticals were developed, Americans became increasingly dependent on physicians for access to improved treatments. Physicians increasingly became the gatekeepers to health care as well as its principal providers.

Physicians gained additional economic power in the second half of the twentieth century. Medicaid and Medicare were enacted and implemented in the mid-1960s. Soon thereafter, third-party payments became more dominant. By sending their bills to someone other than their patients, physicians were able with the passage of time to increase their charges. Thus, physicians gained economic power in addition to enhanced professional status. The medical profession in the United States was arguably able to evolve the way it did because there was no other large group of health care practitioners in a position to challenge them. The only possible challenge to physicians might have come from nurses, but nurses had always assumed a role subservient to that of physicians. Throughout most of history, nursing was not recognized as a profession. Before the twentieth century nurses were either untrained workers or members of a religious order that sought to provide humane treatment to the sick and injured.

In 1860, Florence Nightingale established nursing as a profession in England. The first nursing schools in the United States were established in 1873. They initially met with opposition, but the benefits of trained nurses soon became apparent. The effectiveness of nursing was emphasized in World War I, at which time nurse volunteers gained in the public's esteem because of their patriotism and their services to the Armed Services. The role of the nurse was idealized because of their being dedicated to assisting the sick and further strengthened because of the additional appeal of their deferential behavior towards physicians. This idealized role of the deferential nurse was compatible with the role of the dominant physician. Thus, the further independence of the nursing profession was sidetracked. It became increasingly clear that physicians were not willing to give up their dominant position the more so since such action could adversely affect their future livelihood.

An early example of how physicians acted to protect their own interests can be seen in the 1905 trial of the midwife Hanna Porn in Gardner, Massachusetts. Hanna Porn was a successful midwife, with a practice that threatened local physicians. After numerous physician complaints, she was charged with practicing obstetrics without a license. Despite her popularity with the citizens of Gardner, she was eventually sent to prison in 1909. Incidentally, her practice tripled during the years of her trials, clearly enraging physicians that were all too eager to testify against her.

It should be noted that there were practicing midwives in the United States at the time of Hanna Porn's trials that were not brought up on charges, but these midwives were not perceived to be a threat to most physicians. For example, a midwife that served the poor black population in the South was not perceived to be a threat to most physicians who cared mostly for white people. Henna Porn herself continued to practice after she got out of prison, but by then her practice was too small to be perceived as a threat. No further charges were brought against her.

Physicians in America have maintained their dominance over health care for most of the twentieth century. Other health care professions, such as nurses, remained subservient to them in order to be accepted into the mainstream health care workforce. Groups, such as the American Medical Association (AMA), have long opposed the greater independence of nurses. This largely reflects physicians' new concerns over the growth of nurse practitioners. It should be noted that physicians have shown less resistance to physician assistants. This is primarily due to the willingness of physician assistants to practice under the supervision of a physician, something nurse practitioners sought to break free from.

This last point is critical. Physicians have traditionally not been opposed to other health care professions so long as they operated under their professional control. In 1969, amidst a national perception of a serious physician shortage, the AMA invited nurses to expand their roles by becoming physician assistants. In February of 1970, the AMA executive director, Ernest Howard, made public an AMA plan to help 100,000 nurse become physician assistants. This was to be accomplished in physician offices through personal preceptorships. The nurse would be allowed to have responsibility for direct patient care, including house calls, to the degree that the physician judged it desirable or necessary. The physician would charge under a fee for service arrangement for the nurse's services and would then reimburse her. The AMA, however, had failed to consult the nurses themselves and the reception of their plan was anything but welcomed. In an April 4, 1970 statement, the president of the American Nursing Association (ANA), Dorothy Cornelius stated:

"The ANA board of directors deplores the kind of unilateral decision made by the AMA, since it is not the prerogative of the AMA to speak for any other profession." She went on to object to the AMA'S attempts, as she saw them, to "meet the physician shortage by compounding the shortage of nurses."

Nevertheless, nursing was taken by surprise. Only a month later, dissenting voices began to be heard. The University of Pennsylvania Dean of Nursing, Dorothy Mereness, without breaking completely with Dorothy Cornelius's statements, stated in a speech: "In spite of the misgivings of their colleagues, many graduate nurses will most certainly be interested in relating themselves to a physician and accepting whatever extra training he may deem necessary..." It was only a matter of time until the two professions started bilateral discussions. Representatives from the ANA and the NLN, the two professional groups representing nursing and the AMA, got together to discuss the professions' congruent roles. They formed a committee, which a year later evolved into a number of Joint Practice Commissions. Indeed, within the year, many previous differences were identified or eliminated and after the Nixon administration committed federal funds to the education of physician assistants, it was only a matter of time until their numbers began to increase. Following Nixon's Health Message in 1971, he called for $15 million for the training of physician assistants. Congress passed the Comprehensive Health Manpower Training Act of 1971, part of which explicitly committed federal funds for such training. The Health Training Improvement Act of 1970 and the Nurse Training Act of 1971 also provided additional funding for nurse assistants.

The administration and the Congress were persuaded by the potential that this new hybrid profession presented. Six major promises were set out in a white paper presented in 1972. First, it was viewed as a solution to the physician shortage that the country presumably faced. Second, the new positions were seen as a good opportunity for soldiers returning from Vietnam who had had some medical experience but were not able to practice as physicians. Third, educational costs were expected to decrease since the new professionals would be trained in a much shorter time. Fourth, health expenditures were expected to be moderated since non-physicians would provide care and treatment for less than physicians would charge. Fifth, it was expected that conditions of providing care would improve since non-physicians would spend more time with patients. Finally, a better overall effect would be achieved because non-physicians would promote prevention. Some of these expectations, as we have seen, were not realized. National health expenditures skyrocketed, and educational costs did the same. Furthermore, the physician shortage turned into the threat of a surplus and we are still not certain why physicians continue to see their levels of income continue to rise if there is a surplus of providers. In terms of the last two promises, non-physicians have to a great degree fulfilled expectations.

The evolution of non-physician clinicians was destined one day to raise the issue of autonomous practice, however, when the nurses who sought independence from physicians (especially nurse practitioners), even the nursing profession itself demonstrated some opposition. For example, many situations have been reported where hospital nurses have verbally challenged, questioned, or even ignored the recommendations of a nurse practitioner. Also, there is the example of the midwife Janet Leigh in Boston. After an umbilical cord prolapsed at a birth she attended in 1982, a dispute developed with emergency workers over the management of the emergency. As a result, the Board of Registration in Nursing revoked her license on the grounds of "gross misconduct." This occurred despite expert testimony in favor of Janet Leigh. Clearly, the physician dominance of health care was so strong, at least in some locations, that nurses themselves helped to enforce it. For nurses to gain their independence, they would have to wait for the physician hold over health care to weaken appreciably.

A Different Approach to Health Care

Nurse practitioners, physician assistants, and certified nurse midwives were originally intended to act as physician substitutes. Certified nurse midwifes were first trusted to bring obstetrical care to women in rural Kentucky via the Frontier Nursing Service as early as 1925. Their training today is more narrowly focused than that of NPs and PAs but is bounded by the same principles. It focuses on family planning, gynecology and antepartum, intrapartum and postpartum care. However, certified nurse midwives approach gynecology from a holistic perspective. As we noted, the NP and PA professions were established in the 1960s, when there was a perceived shortage of physicians in primary care, especially in rural areas, as more and more physicians were entering the specialties. The NP was the nursing profession's solution to the problem. The NP was trained to provide primary care within the context of nursing. Most nurse practitioners hold graduate degrees, and current standards require a Master's level degree. NPs are trained in primary care areas such as adult health, family health, gerontology, or pediatrics. As with nursing training, so with nurse practitioners, wellness care and the management of acute and chronic care across a wide spectrum of disease, with a special effort focused on patient education and a case-by-case approach is the educational standard. Likewise, the PA was the medical profession's solution to the shortage, trained to provide primary care usually in conjunction with physicians. Despite this difference, the training for both professions is quite similar.

As the disciplines evolved over time, the three professions were valued for their ability to substitute for physicians in many situations and complement physicians' services with nurses who pursued a holistic approach. By holistic, we mean that NPCs have the skills and training to counsel patients on a wide variety of health promotion issues. These issues include health education for the patient and the patient's family, at-home care for the patient, engagement in self-directed care, preventive health measures, and access to community health resources. These are unique skills that are not covered in standard medical training, but they are covered in the training of NPCs. For this reason, NPCs are not considered to be physician substitutes.

Physicians and non-physician clinicians take different approaches to dealing with patients. Various studies have shown that NPs and PAs are more likely than physicians to spend additional time talking to patients. As a result, they often provide the patient with more and better information. Studies focused exclusively on NPs have shown that NPs are more willing to recommend treatments to fit the patient's lifestyle, increasing the likelihood of compliance. Additional studies have shown that NPs are less likely to prescribe medications than are physicians. As for the midwives, they are taught to regard child-birth as a natural process and not a medical procedure. Thus, they are less inclined to use obstetric devices or undertake a caesarean section. Findings such as these have demonstrated the usefulness of NPCs. At the same time, it would be a mistake to believe that NPCs alone can provide the full range of clinical care. That is to say, a team approach between the more thoroughly trained physician and the NPC is desirable, even necessary. Within such a team approach, NPCs could practice independently from physicians and yet at the same time coordinate their efforts. Educational reforms by health professional schools as well as institutional reforms by insurance companies and hospital administrations could facilitate such a team approach.

There is mounting evidence to suggest that NPCs do have the capability to practice independently of physicians. The most striking example involves midwives. In most countries of Western Europe, midwives attend 70 percent to 100 percent of natural births, while they attend only 8.5 percent of natural births in the United States. If midwives were not as capable as physicians, the European percentages could not be explained.

Similar evidence has been compiled to support the abilities of NPs and PAs. Dean Mary Mundinger of Columbia's School of Nursing points out that virtually every study conducted to assess a NP's ability to provide primary care has shown that NPs provide care equal or superior to that provided by physicians. Additionally, studies have shown that patients who rely on NPs to provide primary care have been satisfied with their services. Less extensive research and anecdotal evidence also support patient satisfaction with and respect for the competence of PAs. Such findings suggest that the real obstacle to the establishment of independent practice is not a lack of competence on the part of the NPCs but institutional constraints ranging from physicians' misconceptions about NPCs that stem from their educational experiences to institutional bias which favor high level specialized treatments. Such constraints and misconceptions, however, are changing.

Today nurse specialists such as NPs, BAs, and CNMs are assuming a less subservient role to physicians. They are being granted more and more independence due both to the economic advantages they offer and their holistic approach to patient care. Despite the benefits associated with their utilization, achieving the ability to practice independently from physicians will not be possible if physicians continue to dominate health care in the way they once did.

The physician dominance of health care came to an end with the rise to prominence of managed care in the 1990s. This event occurred as a result of excessive over-spending for health care in the 1970s and 1980s. With the spread of managed care, the third-party payer system started to phase out. It was replaced by cost sharing between physicians and the managed care providers. Additionally, managed care companies often had the final say over the physician's approach to patient treatment. Thus, physicians were no longer in full control of health care. In their attempt to provide cost effective care to members, managed care companies started to utilize or considerably expand their use of NPs, PAs, and CNMs as physician substitutes.

Clearly, financial incentives exist to utilize more NPs, PAs, and CNMs. The cost of educating a nurse specialist is one-third to one-fourth the cost of educating a physician. In addition, NPs and PAs usually charge lower fees than physicians for providing the same services. As a result, NPs and PAs earn on average one-third the salary of a primary care physician. Home-births attended by a CNM can reduce the cost of a normal childbirth by 66 percent. However, such differences standing alone mean little. The real challenge is to coordinate the production and utilization of both physicians and NPCs. Otherwise we end up with more of both, with an end result of higher total costs. To the extent that the total money flowing into the health care system continues to grow, the market cannot be expected to drive out inefficient providers, be they physicians or NPCs.

Not forgetting the previous point, the approach to patient care taken by NPCs can offer both an economic advantage and a quality advantage. Through counseling, an NPC can help patients achieve a healthier life. This will hopefully prevent or control illness, thus limiting future patient contact with the health care sector. It is important for NPCs that this fact be recognized. If it is not, health care payers (both government and insurance companies) may prefer to utilize only physicians over non-physicians if or when physicians lower their fees.

For optimal health care, it is important that each discipline (physician and non-physician) be recognized and utilized for what it can best offer. Findings indicate that many people are still unaware of who exactly NPCs are, or if they know, many have never been exposed to their services. For this to change, strategies to educate the public about the capabilities of each discipline are necessary.

It should be emphasized that NPCs cannot replace physicians. The scientific knowledge possessed by physicians is necessary in many cases especially when inpatient acute care or outpatient surgical procedures are required, but there are other situations where the services of non-physicians are or may be more appropriate. These situations involve patients with identified risks, chronic diseases, or persons who want to be educated about their future role in maintaining their own health. For optimal health care, a team effort is required. Physicians cannot dominate health care. They have to assume a role where they work in conjunction with non-physician providers for the broader benefit of patients. This is indeed possible. In a recent study about physician perceptions of the nurse practitioner in the 1990s, the authors state, "Physicians who have worked with NPs had a more positive attitude toward the role of the NP and the NP's ability to enhance the provision of primary care services than those who had no direct experience." The obvious implication of such findings has to do with the training of NPCs and physicians. More interdisciplinary training may be one way of enhancing mutual understanding among the different professions and, in turn, build mutual respect, which is the prerequisite for more efficient and effective team outcomes.

The Future Supply of Non-Physician Clinicians

Even a cursory look at recent trends indicates that NPCs are increasing both in absolute numbers and in numbers relative to physicians. Furthermore, a growing number of states are granting different NPC groups professional autonomy that they had not enjoyed until very recently. What is missing is a coordinated policy effort both in terms of the training and the supply of future medical professionals (both physicians and NPCs) and in terms of where and how these professionals will practice.

As table 6.1 shows, the number of traditional NPCs that graduate annually more than doubled between 1992 and 1997, and at the end of 2001 a further increment of 20 percent is projected. Interestingly, the greatest concentrations of NPCs can be found in the same areas with large concentrations of physicians, an oversupply that does not do much to moderate physician maldistribution. Even though the physician assistant movement (out of which the NPCs grew) began in the 1970s as a response to the geographic maldistribution of physicians, most PAs practice in large metro areas as table 6.2 shows. That is not to say that they do not moderate physician maldistribution in rural areas, at least to a limited degree; 20 percent of PAs practice in rural areas. That in itself is significant. An impressive projection is that on a per capita basis, the growth in NPC supply between 1995 and 2005 will be double that of physicians. Table 6.1 shows NPC graduates by year and specialty. Table 6.2 shows clinically active physician assistants by location for 1997.

In terms of the clinical autonomy that NPCs enjoy, the situation varies greatly depending on the state and on the concentration of NPCs in that state, in addition to other key factors. At most, NPCs enjoy, as Cooper, Henderson, and Dietrich put it in a 1998 *JAMA* article, "high degree of autonomy and a broad range of authority to provide discrete levels of uncomplicated and specialty care. States grant practice prerogatives, such as licensure, scope of practice, prescriptive authority, overall autonomy for instance, through different regulations, statutes, and other means. Five major trends in relation to NPCs as autonomous providers of patient care emerge from a review of the literature. First, as mentioned earlier, there is significant variability in the range of prerogatives granted by states to the different NPC groups. Second, the more extensive the prerogatives granted by the state, the more independence NPCs enjoy in that state. Third, NPCs as of today provide a range of services that Cooper calls "simple general care and routine licensed specialty care." Fourth, the extent of NPCs practices is becoming better and more clearly defined every year as more states look into this issue and as market dynamics continue to shape what the states can expect NPCs to perform. Finally, as the increasing numbers of NPCs and as the projec-

Table 6.1
Traditional Non-Physician Clinician Graduates

Year	Nurse Practitioners	Physician Assistants	Certified Nurse Midwives
1992	1500	1360	110
1993	1750	1450	185
1994	2525	1950	235
1995	3600	2150	290
1996	4800	2550	370
1997	6350	2800	414
1998	6600	3100	480
1999	6850	3300	550
2000	7100	3400	600
2001	7250	3400	600

Table 6.2
Clinically Active PAs by Location (percent total)

Large Metro	47.1
Small Metro	33.5
Rural	19.4

tions of their future numbers have already indicated, the more independence NPCs are granted the more students are likely to enter these disciplines. In short, NPCs both as a group but also as individual providers, at the micro level of patient care, are increasing their prerogatives of independence and numbers. Therefore, a more coordinated policy by educators, policymakers, and market actors to ensure better coordination among the different professional providers in U.S. health care is needed, otherwise further fragmentation of the already pluralistic health care system can be expected to lead to further increases in health care expenditures without helping to resolve issues of access and quality of care.

NPs and CNMs are recognized as licensed in all states with the exception of Illinois where legislation is pending. PAs are recognized in all states except Mississippi. Furthermore, traditional non-physician clinicians are allowed to practice independently in twenty-one states. In some states, non-physician clinicians are required to maintain a relationship with a physician, with various states dealing with this issue differently. NPCs can prescribe non-controlled drugs in a third of the states. In the other states, they can prescribe controlled drugs as long as they adhere to certain limitations about the duration of the prescription. Traditional NPCs also enjoy a wide scope of practice. They can in most states perform physicals, order lab tests and interpret them, and perform immunizations. In a few states, they are allowed to perform more invasive procedures like lumbar punctures.

In terms of financing of services, NPCs who work with a physician can charge Medicare and Medicaid. As their independence increases, however, additional approaches will be needed. Some of these became available as early as 1977 under the Rural Health Clinics Act, when, as part of the federal efforts to staff rural clinics NPCs were allowed to charge the government directly without physician supervision. This has since been expanded to cover other sites as well, and unless a state requires a physician's signature, it is not a requirement. Under the Balanced Budget Act of 1997, direct reimbursement by Medicare was extended to NPCs in all non-hospital sites. Almost all states reimburse NPCs through Medicaid, but the rates range from as low as 50 percent of physician services all the way up to 100 percent.

As the previous discussion indicates, the increasing penetration of NPCs into the U.S. health care delivery system is a result both of their increased capabilities and of the increased opportunities they are given to exercise these capabilities. Part of the reason behind these increased opportunities are comparative economic advantages that payers see in NPCs providing care that subspecialist physicians shun or were not trained to provide. Legal barriers to the independent practice of NPCs, however, still exist. In particular, non-physician clinicians are to a great extent limited in their abilities to prescribe medications. Very often, physician approval is required for prescriptions for select or all medications. The specifics vary, as we have seen, from state to state.

As NPCs continue to fight for their independence, physicians fight to maintain their hold over the health care sector. As noted earlier, the AMA (and other physician groups) continues to lobby for NPC to practice under their supervision, thus supporting restrictive laws. NPCs stress their usefulness in providing health care and the need for them to practice independently. Since the number of NPCs in practice increases each year, they have a growing voice in issues concerning health care. They are using this growing voice to speak out against restrictive laws. They know that unless these laws are modified or eliminated, physicians will always have the final say, maintaining their dominance in health care.

As time passes, it seems likely that NPCs will achieve the right to practice independently of physicians. This is due to the economic advantages associated with their use, their competence as providers, and the inability of physician to maintain their dominant position in health care. Still, physicians are a necessary component of health care. Coordination of health care services between physicians and non-physicians will result in an increased quality of health care that will benefit patients.

7

A Look Ahead to 2030

The beginning of the twenty-first century found that the number of allopathic physicians had increased from around 468,000 in 1980 to approximately 768,000 at century's end, or a gain of approximately two-thirds during the two decades, with a doubling in the number of osteopathic physicians during these same two decades from under 20,000 to close to 40,000. Despite these sizable increases in the physician supply over these two decades the total health workforce grew at an even faster rate so that physicians at the century's end accounted for no more than 1 out of every 12 health care workers. The combination of the personnel trends with the demographic aging of the population means that both acute but also chronic care will have to be delivered through different modes including other clinicians in addition to physicians.

Oddly enough, as the 1990s ended and the new decade began, most physician supply issues that had surfaced earlier—such as the prospective shortage of physicians; the excessive proportion of specialists; the maldistribution as between large metropolitan centers and rural areas; the underrepresentation of blacks and Hispanics entering the practice of medicine; the inadequate numbers of physicians available to treat many local populations, especially in low-income urban and in sparsely settled rural areas and of course the relations among physicians, nurses, and other professionals, had for the most part dropped off the national health agenda. The only issue of potential policy significance that seemed to be of any concern to important physician groups, such as the leadership of the American Association of Medical Colleges, the AMA, and the Osteopathic Profession, was for Congress to take early action to reduce the number of IMGs admitted to the United States from around 30 percent of the graduates of U.S. medical schools to no more than 10 percent, a recommendation based on their belief that the United States already faced or would soon face a surplus of physicians, which, if not relieved by reducing the prospective numbers of IMGs, would sooner rather than later force a prospective closure of a considerable number of U.S. medical schools. But so far, Congress has not seen fit to follow this advice because, among other reasons, of the important role that IMGs play in selected states and locations in providing a disproportionate amount of the medical care that recent immigrants, other underserved persons, and many of the poor receive. Simply put, Congress appears to think that even if the requested changes were to be made, the effects would be marginal in terms of the overall supply of physicians. And in light of the IMG services to poorer communities, Congress is not about to jeopardize these services in order to satisfy certain interests of organized medicine. Where does this leave us? What issues are likely to be on the physician supply agenda in the coming decades?

If the critical issue of the future total supply of physicians has been largely removed from the nation's health care agenda, what questions remain that invite early attention and action? Without attaching any special significance to the ordering of the issues noted below, the following have on the one hand been on the agenda of important and concerned health care analysts. Even though the government is not preoccupied with them at this juncture, they are likely to return to the agenda in one form or another.

1.   As we noted earlier in chapter 2, the 3,000 goal of admissions to allopathic medical schools by the year 2000 advocated by the American Association of Medical Colleges fell considerably short at century's end. The shortage cannot be lightly dismissed in face of the radical changes that lie ahead in the differentially rapid growth of both the black and Hispanic population in the first half of the new century, when the estimated total U.S. population will consist of about 40 percent "minorities," with Hispanics, blacks, and Asians accounting for the vast majority. There is a widespread belief among health care analysts that minority groups, and more particularly foreign-speaking minority groups, have considerable health gains to make by obtaining access to and being treated by physicians who speak their native tongue and are well acquainted with their traditions and patterns of living.

2.   Although it is not difficult in 2000 to foresee the changes that may emerge in the years ahead in increasing the decision-making power of physicians, in collaboration with their patients, to determine treat-

ment plans without cancellation or radical modification by unilateral action of their insurance plan, it does not follow that physicians will not be forced to operate within a system of cost constraints although the mechanisms for such constraints still remain to be formulated, accepted, and implemented.

3.   A growing number of professional certifying and licensing groups have been calling attention these last years to the critical importance for medical schools and teaching hospitals to expand by an order of magnitude the role of ambulatory training in the preparation of tomorrow's medical students and residents. While most faculty members are aware of this recommendation and a considerable number have sought to respond to this advice the additional supervisory costs entailed by a radical expansion in ambulatory site training has slowed the wholehearted acceptance of this recommendation. And it is questionable, given the competing demands for "scarce" medical dollars how much progress will be made along this front in the near-middle term.

4.   The foregoing dilemma of finding the additional funding for expanding ambulatory site training warrants a reference to the article authored by Robert Ebert and Eli Ginzberg in the supplement of *Health Affairs*, 1988, which advanced a proposal whereby two years in the current seven-year combined program of medical school and initial board certification could be reorganized to save two years, or 28 percent of the total cost of the currently in place training program. Since the long-in-place, ever more costly U.S. health care system must sooner or later confront the realities of a more constrained financial environment and since the accelerated movement to more ambulatory care training is broadly supported even if it is being only slowly implemented because of cost constraints, a number of cost-saving alternatives including the Ebert-Ginzberg proposal should be reassessed and implemented, at least in part if not in whole.

While on the subject of potential cost-savings to facilitate alternative expenditures, one cannot overlook the fact that acute care hospital occupancy nationwide is in the low 60 percent range, and in selected locations in the 50 and even in the 40 percent range. Admittedly, there is nothing easy about merging or closing surplus hospital capacity in the face of trustee responsibilities for hospital debt; the dependence of neighboring populations on local hospital care; the importance of the community hospital in providing jobs and income to many of the local workforce, and for still other reasons. But if the U.S. Armed Forces have found it possible to close a large number of surplus establishments, the challenge of shrinking the acute care hospital infrastructure, especially with the assistance of the federal and state governments, should not continue to be ignored, even if constructive resolutions will prove difficult to design and implement.

6.   The challenge to resize the acute care hospital sector is that much more pressing once one takes cognizance of the growing numbers of the elderly suffering from one or more chronic conditions who live at home, or in an assisted living arrangement in their community, preferring if at all possible not to enter a nursing home for a shorter or longer stay with an annual charge of around $40,000 and considerably more for a year's stay at a well-appointed facility, for which most seniors have no insurance coverage and must be Medicaid eligible or rely on family funds.

7.   One must quickly note that home care and the financing thereof is not free of serious challenges. Witness the turmoil created by Medicare's rapid cutback in its home health benefits after the passage of the Balanced Budget Act of 1997. The United States confronts a number of challenges for improving the care of patients with chronic illness living at home. Consider the following:

•   Will physicians, specialists, or generalists alter their half-century and longer failure to make home visits? The answer is not likely because as noted earlier physicians are increasingly dependent on the use of increasingly sophisticated diagnostic and curative technology. Two further observations are critical: it is very costly in terms of the physicians' time and energy to visit patients in their homes, the more so if the patient is capable of coming to the office, clinic, or hospital. And while certain patients may have little or no mobility it does not follow that they must be seen by a physician, surely not routinely. As noted in the preceding chapter, the last several years have seen a marked increase in the number of nurse practitioners and other NPCs who, working as members of a larger team of health professionals, including one or more physicians, are able to assume most of the responsibility for home visits to assess and provide at least basic care for the home bound patient. Admittedly, some chronic patients are more or less immobile and would require transportation to a hospital or clinical center for more elaborate work-up, assessment, or treatment.

•   While some efforts have been made by selected medical schools and teaching hospitals to put in place training programs in which physicians have the opportunity to gain experience as a member of a team of clinicians and therapists with shared responsibility for patient care, one must quickly add that such joint training and operations remain more theory than reality. Most physicians see themselves as the medical leadership profession and are disinclined to enter into a shared team responsibility for patient care with non-physician clinicians.

The United States confronts two remaining challenges. What lessons can be drawn from our review of physician supply policies as a key to improved health care delivery to the American people during the last third of the twentieth century? And what are the prospects that further attention to physician supply policies will be able to improve the efficiency and effectiveness of the U.S. health care delivery system during the first third of the twenty-first century.

Three related developments on the physician supply front emerged during the last decade and a half of the twentieth century that seem critical to the future developments of medical personnel supply. It appeared for a time that the market demand would result in reducing the number of young physicians preparing for a specialist career in favor of general practice, but before the century's end much of the momentum for such a shift had dissipated as more and more Medicare as well as other patients resented having to get clearance from the generalist physician in order to revisit the specialist who had been treating them.

Second, the leading medical professional and medical educational bodies became increasingly concerned about the substantial increase in the numbers of IMGs who were being admitted to the United States for residency training, but despite continuing lobbying on their part Congress refused to alter this inflow, among other reasons because the legislators recognized that IMGs in selected states such as New York, New Jersey, Connecticut, Michigan, and a few others depended very heavily on IMGs to help care for large numbers of low-income patients who lived in areas that the graduates of U.S. medical schools tended to avoid.

And thirdly, with nurse practitioners in the lead a number of non-physician clinical providers assumed ever more responsibility for providing care for ever larger numbers of low-income patients, especially many who were suffering from chronic conditions and were living at home and often sought treatment in nearby clinics.

The final question that we need to address, informed by the overall expansion of the last third of the twentieth century and the three main developments that we have just discussed, is whether and how federal and state governments and the considerable number of medical schools under non-profit auspices should place physician supply policies high on their policy agenda during the first third of the twenty-first century?

Let us note at the beginning of our answer that we believe that the federal government, in close partnership with many state governments, was justified in its 1960-70 effort to seek and achieve what turned out to be a doubling, essentially, of the physician supply per

100,000 population, from roughly 140 in the early 1960s to 280 at century's end. Even with this substantially increased supply, gross differences persist in the number of physicians per 100,000 available to Americans of the order of five-fold, depending on where they live, their income levels, and their hospital infrastructure. One must also keep the following in perspective: In the absence of a war, or mobilization for a war, the United States will not interfere with the rights of the individual to pursue the career of his or her choice as well as the location where he or she will practice when their studies have been completed.

Two related considerations: the number of fully qualified students seeking admission to U.S. medical schools continues to exceed current capacity; and a review of physicians' earnings shows that with a single exception (1994) there has been a steady upward trend with the average approximating at the beginning of 2001, $200,000 net.

In short, this preliminary reading suggests that there is no basis, surely no strong basis, for early and strong action by the governmental and non-profit sectors, individually or collectively, to initiate policies aimed at reducing the number of physicians who will be entering practice in the years ahead.

A review of the so-called specialist-generalist imbalance that has received considerable attention during the past two decades also reinforces the conclusion that "the future management" of the physician supply is easier to formulate than to implement, given the right of the individual to decide on his or her career preference. It has long been recognized by informed insiders that the gross descriptors of "generalist" and "specialist" may often obscure as much as they reveal. A large and probably growing number of specialists act as the "generalist physician" to many of their patients who are afflicted with one or more chronic diseases, an arrangement that has developed because it makes sense to both parties.

At the beginning of the twenty-first century, there are a few projections about the changing needs and demands of the U.S. population for medical care, up to twenty or thirty that can be developed with reasonable assurance; and there are many others that remain hidden even to the leaders of the profession. Among the high priority challenges that are not likely to disappoint will be a doubling of the elderly population above 65, and a corresponding large increase in the numbers of Americans who will live into their eighties and even nineties. But having identified this trend in the future need/demand for medical care one must quickly add that in the absence of truly heroic advances in medical treatment a high proportion of the much enlarged elderly group will be suffering from one or more chronic conditions; and, for the most part, they will be living at home or in their communities in assisted living arrangements.

If past is prologue, and it may turn out not to be, caregivers will be paid employees who help with shopping, cooking, bathing, and otherwise assisting the chronically ill elderly. There may be a nurse practitioner who visits on occasion to assess whether the patient is being well cared for and to provide some not too complicated medical or pharmaceutical interventions. If the patient develops an acute condition he or she is likely to be assisted to visit a physician in an office, clinic, or hospital for more definitive assessment and treatment. An article entitled "Long-Term Care for the Elderly with Disabilities" by Robyn I. Stone, recently published by the Milbank Fund, argues that the United States has a grossly inadequate number of geriatricians. But in reaching this conclusion the author fails to disclose the basis for such a conclusion; and further, fails to point to ways that the so-called "shortage" can be relieved. Our family physician of a half-century ago was a specialist in internal medicine, but the bulk of his practice was centered on caring for his above 65-year-old patients.

We return once again to our basic question: to what extent should the U.S. providers of health care, the leaders of medical education, and the leaders of the medical profession focus attention on physician policy changes in the hope and expectation that these initiatives will lead to significant gains in increasing the efficiency of the medical care system and improving patient outcomes with special attention to the growing subgroup of vulnerable patients, the elderly, particularly those above 75 years of age. With most of the elderly living at home or in the community, there are a number of challenges that, if addressed and met, such as the training and supervision of the basic workforce of paraprofessionals and improvement of their levels of pay, hold greater promise than seeking to fine tune the supply.

But the challenges of providing effective care to the chronically ill in their own homes present policymakers with a number of further difficulties. Number 7 of the Profiles released by the National Academy on an Aging Society (on "Caregiving") makes the following introductory points: Two out of five people over 70 need help with one or more daily activities. Yet many do not receive the care they need. For example, more than one-third of elderly people who live in a community have unmet daily activities needs.

The majority of the elderly who do receive help rely on family and friends. In 1997, unpaid caregivers provided care worth an estimated $196 billion. The significance of this last figure can be judged by the fact that it accounted for about one out of every five dollars of NHE in that year.

Spouses provided between 28 percent and 35 percent of the care that white, black and Hispanic patients received and the children and grandchildren of the three groups provided, respectively 45 percent, 52 percent, and 58 percent of the required care.

Moreover, some 8.5 million persons over the age of 70 have limitations with activities of daily living (ADL), such as using the toilet, getting out of bed, driving or walking; or institutional activities of daily living (IADL), such as taking medications, preparing meals, or managing their money. While only 37 percent of the 70+ population report their physical health status to be fair or poor, for those with IADLs, 60 percent report their health status to be fair or poor; and for those with ADLs the numbers rise to 63 percent. By the year 2030, the number of people aged 70+ needing care is projected to more than double to 21 million, up from 10 million in 2000.

All these trends have affected tremendously and adversely the health not only of the patients but also of their current caregivers. This adds considerably to the unsolved problems that confront the United States at the beginning of the twenty-first century and are almost certain to worsen as the number of the elderly population doubles in the coming third of a century. A considerable number (30 percent) of women caregivers currently report being emotionally strained with another 30 percent reporting physical or mental health problems or physical strain. Not a good augury for what lies ahead.

Judith Feder and her colleagues Harriet L. Kiomisar and Marlene Nufeld characterized the long-term care system in an article in *Health Affairs*, May-June 2000, entitled "Long-Term Care in the United States: An Overview" as: "A complex system of public and private funding often leaves elderly persons at risk of financial catastrophe and inadequate care." This is a description that is hard to challenge once one reads through their analysis and assesses their conclusions. One might caution that with so many problems in the areas of acute care that remain unsolved including the 42 million persons in the United States without health insurance coverage it should come as no surprise, or at least as no big surprise, that the unsolved health care and maintenance support problems of the elderly living at home present an equally if not more serious type of neglect. It should be noted that Germany recently provided compulsory insurance coverage for the long-term care of the elderly, including payments to family members who volunteer to provide such care to their frail elderly living at home. But most advanced nations have left all or most of the responsibility to the immediate family for caring for their weak and disabled elderly relatives.

It is not only difficult but well nigh impossible to outguess in the year 2003 the policies that the United States will consider as well as those that it will seek to implement in the decades ahead when the numbers of the frail elderly living at home are likely to double; and when a growing proportion of them will be in their eighties or nineties, with growing numbers of centenarians. One assumption, however, can be safely ventured: sooner and surely later the United States will have to confront this largely ignored challenge; and even if its political leaders and the public are very supportive and responsive the country is likely to encounter many difficulties before finding answers that the majority of the voters will accept and approve.

The United States cannot respond effectively to the prospectively larger numbers of elderly persons, many of whom will be capable of continuing to be employed, some full-time and more part-time surely up to age 80, and a considerable minority even longer, without tackling and at least beginning to solve the multiple changes in its long established practices that led most individuals to retire in their early mid-sixties. A society can face, as the United States is likely to face, the enforced retirement of an ever larger proportion of its adult population twenty years before it loses the capacity to be productively engaged. But no society will find it easy to address and resolve even some, if not all, of the complex issues affecting changes in the conventional age of retirement, private and publicly supported health care programs such as Medicare Social Security payments, and a host of other complex laws, regulations, and practices.

But the sooner we begin to recognize that these challenges exist and can only gain momentum with the passage of every year; that they result from the gains in longevity and years of healthy life that our economy and health care programs have made possible; and that the solutions go beyond the capacity of individuals to develop and implement without the full participation of the larger society-government, corporations, nonprofit institutions, religious bodies, the educational system and many more, the search for answers will be delayed and the solutions will prove even more difficult to explore and implement. The full costs of the progress that we have made must be met at least in part before further progress will be possible.

In conclusion, physician supply policies cannot work if the goal is to fix underlining problems that face the U.S. health care system, such as access and cost. Medical personnel supply policy can help the nation's health care system to adjust to the new challenges that technology and demography present it. We do not feel that a trend of physician specialization is threatening if a medical team approach is adopted. It can assist in the major issue of improving the health care for the elderly through establishing connections between all levels of care, preventive, acute, and chronic.

Selected Reading

Books

Bodenheiiner, T. S., and K. Grumbach. *Understanding Health Policy: A Clinical Approach.* Stamford, Conn.: Appleton and Lange, 1995.

Campion, Frank D. *The AMA and US Health Policy Since 1940.* Chicago: Chicago Review Press, 1984.

Fuchs, V. *The Health Economy.* Cambridge, Mass.: Harvard University Press, 1986.

Ginzberg, Eli. *Tomorrow's Hospital: A Look to the Twenty-First Century.* New Haven, Conn: Yale University Press, 1996.

Ginzberg, Eli, ed. *Critical Issues in US Health Reform.* Boulder, Colo.: Westview Press, 1994.

Ginzberg Eli. *The Financing of Medical Schools.* Proceedings of a Josiah Macy Jr. Foundation Conference. New York, *1995.*

Ginzberg Eli, Miriam Ostow, and Anna Dutka. *The Economics of Medical Education.* Proceedings of a Josiah Macy Jr. Foundation Conference. New York, 1993.

Ginzberg E., Howard Berliner, and Miriam Ostow. *Improving the Health Care of the Poor: The New York City Experience.* New Brunswick, N.J.: Transaction Publishers, 1997.

Harman, Denham, Robin Holiday, and Mohsen Meydani, eds. *Towards Prolongation of the Healthy Life Span.* Annals of the New York Academy of Sciences, vol. 854. New York, 1998.

Morris, Thomas, and Glenda Garvey. *Taking Charge of Graduate Medical Education: To Meet the Nation's Needs in the 21st Century.* Proceedings of a Josiah Macy Jr. Foundation Conference. New York, 1993.

Starr, Paul. *The Social Transformation of American Medicine.* New York: Basic Books, 1983.

Journals

Academic Medicine
Health Affairs
Health Care Financing Review
Hospital and health Networks
Inquiry
Journal of the American Medical Association

Journal of Health Politics, Policy and Law
Modern Healthcare
New England Journal of Medicine

Articles and Reports

Cohen, J., and M. Whitcomb. "Are the Recommendations of the AAMC 's Task Force on the Generalist Physicians Still Valid?" *Academic Medicine.* Vol. 72(1): 13-16, January 1997.

The Commonwealth Fund Task Force on Academic Health Centers Report. "Leveling the Playing Field: Financing the Missions of Academic Health Centers." New York, May 1997.

Cooper R., P. Laud, and B. S. Dietrich. "Current and Projected Workforce of Nonphysician Clinicians." *JAMA* 280(9): 788-794, September 2, 1998.

Dersan, Lori, and Maggie Fischbusch, eds. "Academic Health Centers and the Community: A Practical Guide for Creating Shared Visions." Health of the Public Program Office, University of California, San Francisco, 1992.

Foreman, S. "The Changing Academic Medical Center." 39th Annual Induction Speech in the NY Chapter of Alpha Omega Alpha, New York, May 5, 1997.

Ginzberg, Eli. "The Future Supply of Physicians." *Academic Medicine* (1996) 71: 1147-1153.

Ginzberg, Eli. "The Changing U.S. Health Care Agenda." *JAMA* 279(7): 501-504, February 18, 1998.

Iglehart, J. K. "Rapid Changes for Academic Medical Centers." *New England Journal of Medicine* (1995) 332: 407-411.

lglehart J. K. "The Quandary Over Graduates of Foreign Medical Schools in the United States." *NEJM* 334 (25): 1679-1683.

Iglehart J. K. "Medicare and Graduate Medical Education" *NEJM* 338 (6): 402-407.

Institute of Medicine. "The Nation's Physician Workforce: Options for Balancing Supply and Requirements." IOM, National Academy Press, Washington D.C., 1996.

Institute of Medicine. "On Implementing a National Graduate Medical Education Trust Fund." IOM, National Academy Press, Washington D.C., 1997.

Jones, R. "Academic Medicine: Institutions, Programs and Issues." Association of American Medical Colleges Report, Washington, D.C., February 1997.

Kassirer, J. P. "Academic Medical Centers Under Siege." *New England Journal of Medicine* (1994) 331: 1370-1371.

Mullan, F., R. M. Politzer, and C. H. Davis. "Medical Migration and the Physician Workforce: International Medical Graduates and American Medicine." *JAMA* (1995) 273: 1521-1527.

Pew Charitable Trusts. "Critical Challenges: Revitalizing the Health Professions for the Twenty-First Century. UCSF Center for the Health Professions Department. San Francisco, 1995.

Reinhardt, U. "Wanted: A Clearly Articulated Social Ethic for American Health Care." *JAMA* 278(17): 1446-l447, November 5, 1997.

Rice, D. P., and C. Hoffman. "Chronic Care in America: A 21st Century Challenge." The Institute for Health and Aging at University of California, San Francisco, and The Robert Wood Johnson Foundation, Princeton, N.J., August 1996.

Rosenbaum, S., K. Maloy, J. Stuber, and J. Darnell. "Initial Findings from a Nationwide Study of Outstationed Medical Enrollment Programs at Federally Qualified Health Centers." The Center for Health Policy Research at George Washington University, Washington, D.C., February 1998.

Rosenblat M., M. Rabkin, and D. Tosteson. "How One Teaching Hospital System and One Medical School are Jointly Affirming Their Academic Mission." *Academic Medicine* 72 (6): 483-488, June 1997.

Ruzek, J., F. O'Neil, R. Willard, and R. W. Rimel. "Trends in U.S. Funding for Biomedical Research." The Center for the Health Professions at UCSF and the Pew Scholars Program in the Biomedical Sciences, San Francisco, May 1996.

Stimmel, B. D. "Congress and the International Medical Graduate: The Need for Equity." *Mt. Sinai Journal of Medicine* (1996) 63: 359-363.

Thorpe, K. E. "The Rising Number of Uninsured Workers: An Approaching Crisis in Health Care Financing." The National Coalition on Health Care, Washington, D.C., October 1997.

Ware, J., M. Bayliss, W. Rogers, M. Kosinski, and A. R. Tarlov. "Differences in 4-year Health Outcomes for Elderly and Poor, Chronically Ill Patients Treated in HMO and Fee for Service Systems." *JAMA* (1996) 276 (13): 1039-1047.

Data Sources

American Hospital Association: Emerging Trends Quarterly Briefs. Chicago, 1993-1998.

Association of American Medical Colleges. AAMC Data Book: Statistical Information Related to Medical Education. Washington, D.C., January 2001.

Council on Graduate Medical Education Reports to Congress and the Secretary of Health and Human Services, 1986-1999.

Graduate Medical Education National Advisory Committee Report (GMENAC). Seven vols. U.S. Department of Health and Human Services, Washington D.C. 1980.

Health Insurance Association of America. Source Book of Health Insurance Data, 1996. Washington, D.C., HIAA, 1997.

Health Systems Research, Inc. "The Development of Capitation Rates Under Medicaid Managed Care Programs: A Pilot Study," Vols. 1 and 2. The Henry J. Kaiser Family Foundation, Washington, D.C., November 1997.

Institute for Health Care Research and Policy. "Medicare Chart Book." The Henry J. Kaiser Family Foundation. Washington, D.C., June 1997.

Medicare Payment Advisory Commission. "Medicare Payment Policy: Report to the Congress, Vol. 1: Recommendations, and Vol. 2: Analytical Papers. Washington, D.C., March 1998.

National Institute for Health Care Management. Health Care System Data Source, second ed. Washington, D.C., NIHCM, July 1998.

Periodic Reports issued by the Congressional Budget Office Dealing with Health Care Current Expenditures and Future Projections. Washington, D.C.

Periodic Reports issued by the General Accounting Office Related to Physician Supply and Medicare and Medicaid Policies. Washington, D.C., 1994-1997.

Periodic Reports from The Center for Health Workforce Studies Related to Physician and Non Physician Clinician Trends in the Country. School of Public Health, SU7NY Albany, Rensselaer, New York.

Physician Payment Review Commission. Annual Report to Congress, 1999. Washington, D.C., 1999.

Physicians: A Study of Physician's Fees. A Report by the Council on Wage and Price Stability, Executive Office of the President. Washington D.C., March 1978.

Physician's Income in the Pre-Medicare Period-1965. A Report by the U.S. Department of Health, Education and Welfare, January 1976.

U.S. Bureau of the Census. Statistical Abstract of the United States: 1999. (119th ed.) Washington, D.C., October 1999.

Index